THE RISK OF A LIFETIME

THE RISK OF A LIFETIME

How, When, and Why Procreation May Be Permissible

Rivka Weinberg

OXFORD
UNIVERSITY PRESS

OXFORD
UNIVERSITY PRESS

Oxford University Press is a department of the University of Oxford.
It furthers the University's objective of excellence in research, scholarship,
and education by publishing worldwide.

Oxford New York
Auckland Cape Town Dar es Salaam Hong Kong Karachi
Kuala Lumpur Madrid Melbourne Mexico City Nairobi
New Delhi Shanghai Taipei Toronto

With offices in
Argentina Austria Brazil Chile Czech Republic France Greece
Guatemala Hungary Italy Japan Poland Portugal Singapore
South Korea Switzerland Thailand Turkey Ukraine Vietnam

Oxford is a registered trade mark of Oxford University Press
in the UK and certain other countries.

Published in the United States of America by
Oxford University Press
198 Madison Avenue, New York, NY 10016

© Oxford University Press 2016

First issued as an Oxford University Press paperback, 2017

Library of Congress Cataloging-in-Publication Data
Weinberg, Rivka.
The risk of a lifetime : how, when, and why procreation may be permissible /
Rivka Weinberg.
p. cm.
Includes bibliographical references and index.
ISBN 978-0-19-024370-8 (hardcover); 978-0-19-069599-6 (paperback)
1. Human reproduction—Moral and ethical aspects. 2. Reproductive rights. I. Title.
HQ766.15.W45 2015
176—dc23
2015003316

To those I forced into existence:
My children,
Rami and Joey
Forgive me. I hope it treats you well.

CONTENTS

ACKNOWLEDGMENTS

I have benefited from comments and discussions with many people on the ideas and arguments developed in this book. For helpful comments and discussion, I am grateful to the late Jonathan Adler, Sonja Alsofi, Elizabeth Anderson, David Benatar, Michael Cholbi, Ann Davis, Jeanine Diller, Zev Gruman, Elizabeth Harman, Peter Kung, Jeff McMahan, Derek Parfit, Melinda Roberts, Peter Singer, Doran Smolkin, David Velleman, Charles Young, and the members of the Claremont Philosophers Work-In-Progress Group. In addition to much helpful discussion, I am deeply grateful to David Boonin, Saul Smilansky, and David Wasserman for written comments on the entire manuscript. I am also especially grateful to Yuval Avnur, for much discussion and many rounds of helpful written comments. All of my philosophical work, including all the work in this book, has benefited immeasurably from innumerable insightful comments on many rounds of drafts, multiple and endless discussions, and largely undeserved encouragement from Paul Hurley and Dion Scott-Kakures. My debt to them is immense, as is my gratitude.

I am grateful to my professors who encouraged me in my early pursuit of philosophy at Brooklyn College, CUNY, including Ed Kent, Beth Singer, and, most especially, Andrew Wengraf and the late Jonathan Adler. And I am grateful to my students who have illuminated these matters in discussion and writing with me, especially Taylor Bouchard, Ilona Phipps-Morgan, Suzie Love, Daniella Urban, and Stephanie Widmer. I thank Scripps College for sabbatical leaves and fellowships that supported this research.

Thanks to audiences at Hebrew University, the Ira W. Decamp Bioethics seminar at Princeton University, the University of Haifa, and the Rocky Mountain Ethics Congress for helpful comments and discussion.

Special thanks to Lucy Randall, Associate Editor at Oxford University Press, for shepherding this manuscript from its infancy through its completion.

For the personal support that enables all of my work, I owe thanks as well to all of my friends, especially the late Jonathan Adler, Michele Beck, Sheldon Londner, Laki Maza, Taaly Silberstein, and Joyce Tamara for their patience, endurance, and support; and to all of my sisters for their support, especially my sister Miriam Perr, my wisest and funniest friend from birth.

If I were grateful for my existence, I might thank my parents for causing my existence, but then I'd have to thank the Protestant and Catholic Churches for European anti-Semitism because I surely would not exist if Hitler and his countless anti-Semitic supporters in Germany and Poland had not caused my grandparents to flee their respective European countries, taking their children with them to the same country, enabling my parents to meet, and conceive me. As it turns out, I'm not very partial to existence, nor am I very grateful for it. I am instead grateful to my parents for their living examples of generosity, integrity, and independence of mind.

I am grateful to my husband, Zev Gruman, whose love, wit, intelligence, and understanding make my life possible. And I am grateful to my children, Rami and Joey, for enriching my life and work with their awesome and fascinating being.

And, finally, thanks to my colleague Peter Kung, for telling me to stop reading and start writing already.

Parts of this book include materials discussed in previously published papers. Thanks to the publishers of *Philosophical Studies* (Springer), *The Journal of Moral Philosophy* (Brill), *Bioethics* (John Wiley & Sons), *Public Affairs Quarterly* (University of Illinois Press), and *South African Journal of Philosophy* (Taylor & Francis) for permission to use this material.

THE RISK OF A LIFETIME

———

Introduction

Everybody is somebody's fault. Everyone who has ever lived is the result of someone else's procreative act (chicken and egg problem aside). If we wish to procreate, we ought to consider our act with the moral seriousness it merits because procreation involves imposing life's risks on whoever will have to live with them. That makes procreation a morally weighty act. This book addresses the central issues in procreative ethics, both theoretical and applied.

Creating people is both an extraordinary and commonplace thing to do. That's an intriguing combination and calls for some reflection. At the outset of the book, in Chapter 1, I analyze the kind of act procreativity is and why we might be justifiably motivated to engage in it, aside from our biological impulse to do so. I argue that procreation is not a gift but is instead a risk imposed on children in order for people to enrich their lives by engaging in the parent-child relationship as a parent. Procreation is not a gift because not only must we work hard if we are to stand a chance at enjoying life, if we don't put in significant effort—and, unfortunately, often even if we do—we will likely endure great suffering. Life is a risk. Perhaps one worth taking and worth imposing, but a risk nonetheless. I argue that whether a particular procreative act is morally acceptable or not depends on the nature of the risk, the likelihood of its ripening into harms or benefits, and the interests people have in imposing it.

Thinking about our interest in procreating involves thinking about procreative motivation. Why do people want to procreate? Procreative motivation is rarely discussed or critically evaluated, yet procreation can seem in tension with our liberal principles of autonomy, consent, and equality. Although we value autonomy and therefore try not to do things that significantly impact others without their consent, we create children entirely without their consent even though creating someone is one of the most impactful things we can ever do to another person. Although we value equality and often strive for equality as an ideal in our interpersonal relationships, the parent-child relationship is inherently unequal for a good deal of the child's life and (even worse) for the time period for which many parents seek it out. Yet there is a nonobjectionable reason for this: people are interested in raising children. The desire to engage in the parent-child relationship as a parent is, I argue, a valid and morally acceptable procreative motivation. Because engaging in the parent-child relationship as a parent is very valuable to parents and can be fulfilling to children as well, the desire to engage in the parent-child relationship as a parent is a morally palatable procreative motivation and one that, I argue, plausibly accords with human experience.

I then turn to questions of procreative permissibility. First, in Chapter 2, I clarify who needs to be concerned about procreative permissibility, that is, who is (morally) parentally responsible. I argue that by virtue of our ownership and control of the hazardous material that is our gametes, we are parentally responsible for the risks we take with our gametes and for the persons that develop when we engage in activity that allows our gametes to unite with others and develop into persons. I call this the Hazmat Theory of parental responsibility and defend it against alternative theories of parental responsibility, including causal, genetic, gestational, and intentional theories, as well as various combinations of these theories. If we accept the Hazmat Theory of parental responsibility, as I argue we should, then it turns out that we are responsible for the children that result from all of our actions that risk allowing our gametes to unite with others and develop into persons. One such action is gamete donation or sale. I argue that this is a credible result that we must face, especially since there is no theory of parental responsibility that will allow us to hold gamete donors/sellers free of parental responsibility yet continue to maintain that accidental parents—people who procreate due to birth control failure, say—are parentally responsible.

Once we know to whom the questions of procreative permissibility apply most directly, I turn to extreme views regarding procreative permissibility, namely, that procreation is almost always permissible and that procreation is almost never permissible. Those are the topics of Chapters 3 and 4, respectively. In Chapter 5, I develop a theory of procreative permissibility, and in Chapter 6, I apply the theory to a wide variety of cases.

In Chapter 3, I consider whether procreation is almost always permissible. This would be the case if the famous non-identity problem were both unsolvable and unavoidable. The non-identity problem asks us who is harmed by acts that seem to involve procreative negligence yet don't seem to harm anyone. For example, if a fourteen-year-old girl wants to procreate, how can we argue that this is contrary to the interests of the child she would have at fourteen? If she delays procreation, she will have a *different* child since it will grow from a different sperm/egg combination, from gametes released years later. So the child she would have at fourteen has only one shot at existence and that shot comes with a fourteen-year-old mother. So long as that child's life is likely to be worth living, overall, according to the non-identity problem we cannot locate any procreative moral wrong. This has been taken by some to imply that nearly all procreativity is permissible since all we need consider is whether the future person's life is likely to be worth living, overall.

I point out that exactly none of our prevailing ethical theories determines moral permissibility on the basis of an act's effects on a particular identifiable individual, so it turns out that the non-identity problem is easily avoided by adopting any of the predominant ethical theories on offer, including Kantian/deontological theories, consequentialist theories, or Aristotelian/virtue ethical theories. So if we can't solve the non-identity problem, following any of our prevailing ethical theories will allow us to avoid its counterintuitive implications.

But I also argue that we need not avoid the problem because there is actually no non-identity *problem*. It is simply a mistake. The mistake, I argue, is the consideration of existence itself, which everyone has and nobody needs, as a good bequeathed to you by your ancestors, that is capable of offsetting or outweighing other life burdens. Existence, I argue, is a prerequisite of being the subject of benefits and burdens, but it is not itself a benefit. It's just a precondition of being subject to benefits and burdens. If we don't count existence itself as a benefit, then we can clearly see that the fourteen-year-old mother burdens her future child with all of the burdens that come along with having a child for a parent. That burden might be offset or outweighed by other life goods that the child manages to secure, but having a teen mother remains a burden inflicted by the teen parent and contrary to the interests of the child. The fact that the child would otherwise not exist at all is of no moral relevance. If you don't exist, you are of no moral relevance, even to yourself. (It's a bit more complicated: you are not a "you" at all; you are a merely possible person, and merely possible people are of no moral relevance.)

Finally, in Chapter 3, I show that deontology can point right at the person wronged by acts of procreative negligence. It can do that because deontology does not require that a person's first-personal interests be set back, overall, in order for a wrong to have been done to that person. Deontology can consider an act wrong because of the way the people involved treat each other, regardless of the consequences.

Since the non-identity problem does not give us near procreative carte blanche, we must take full responsibility for the risk of life our children face. That is no small matter. Life is tough, for almost everyone some of the time and for many people nearly all of the time. So how can we justify procreating?

In Chapter 4, I take up two central lines of argument regarding the general impermissibility of procreativity. The first line of argument analyzes the risk of a lifetime as one that is not worth taking and therefore not permissible to impose. Since most people are glad to be alive and glad to have been born, this line of argument implies that people err in their assessments of their life's value. But how can we know this? Since we all stand equally within life, I argue that there is no more objective place from which to make judgments regarding the general value and quality of human life to the person living it. If people consider their lives valuable and worthwhile, in what way are we better positioned to judge their assessment, and to judge them to be in error? I then consider whether nearly everyone truly has a low quality of life, in terms of hedonistic, desire fulfillment, and objective-list theories of human well-being, and I show that on all of these theories, it is far from clear that most people fare poorly, especially since none of these measures of life's quality ignores the subjective experience and evaluation of the person living the life in question. So long as people seem to love life, it is hard to prove that they are making some kind of objective mistake to do so.

The second line of argument against all procreativity is based on the fact that all people are born without their consent even though it is no harm to anyone not to be born. Since benefits of this type cannot be imposed without prior consent, it is argued, all procreation involves a problematic rights violation. However, I argue that children do not have consent rights since they are not yet competent autonomous agents. Paternalism is justified and appropriate when making decisions that affect children, including decisions that have lifelong effects.

So both lines of argument to the conclusion that procreation is nearly always wrong have very significant flaws. Still, I argue, they do leave us with concerns that cannot be completely assuaged. Some of these concerns include the fact that many people do not find their lives valuable to them and are not glad to have been born. One of those people may be the child you will have. Life is risky for everyone and can entail untold and unremitting suffering, even in cases where that seems initially an unlikely outcome. Forcing people into life, as we do when we procreate, may not sit so easily with those of us who place great value on autonomy, even though we understand that children are not capable of autonomy and don't have consent rights. I conclude that although procreation is probably not always wrong, it remains not only a welfare risk but also a moral risk.

Still, I argue that it is a risk that is sometimes rational and permissible to impose. In Chapter 5, I argue for principles of procreative permissibility directly and independently, as well as on Kantian/Rawlsian contractualist grounds. I begin by arguing for

the use of a Kantian/Rawlsian framework for constructing principles of procreative permissibility. The Kantian framework is suited
to questions of procreative permissibility because it emphasizes
the treatment of all persons as ends in themselves and stresses the
importance of proper motivation. (I argue that procreative motivation is morally very important, in Chapter 1, and its importance
is further underscored by the discussion and arguments in Chapter 4.) The Rawlsian framework is particularly useful for questions
of procreative permissibility because it is constructed to yield just
principles in cases of distributive conflicts of interests and deliber-
ated about under conditions constructed to reduce bias. Although
it is not common to think of procreation as a distributive conflict
of interest kind of case, I argue that it is one: prospective parents
have an interest in procreating whenever they please, and future
children have an interest in excellent birth conditions. These interests are often in conflict. For example, if parents procreate while
they are unemployed, their children will bear some of the costs
of their parents' procreative freedom. If we restrict procreative
permissibility only to cases where the future children are likely
to have extremely secure economic situations, people who cannot
offer this to their children will bear the costs of the security of
future children (a category that, in this case, will not include their
own children).

I then construct the Rawlsian thought experiment as applied
to questions of procreative permissibility. This discussion includes
arguments for the assumption of existence, for an objective list of
basic procreative goods, and for a decision principle that directs
us to maximize our chances of attaining high levels of important procreative goods, while prioritizing the good of self-respect
(since without self-respect, we may be unmotivated to value our
own good). I further argue that the Kantian/Rawlsian framework,

as well as independent considerations of fairness and the ethics of risk imposition, will lead us to the following principles of procreative permissibility:

> *Procreative Balance*: Procreation is permissible only when the risk you impose as a procreator on your children would not be irrational for you to accept as a condition of your own birth (assuming that you will exist), in exchange for the permission to procreate under these risk conditions.
>
> *Motivation Restriction*: Procreation must be motivated by the desire and intention to raise, love, and nurture one's child once it is born.

I then compare my principles to a wide variety of alternate procreative ethical principles, including birthright principles, non-identity principles, eugenic principles (the "best"), procreative liberty principles, strict liability principles, and sanctity-of-life principles, among others. I argue that on their own terms, on Kantian/Rawlsian contractualist grounds, and in comparison to the current procreative ethical theories on offer, the principles I argue for are more fair, more reasonable, and more consistent with the broad moral and legal framework of the ethics of risk imposition than the alternatives.

In Chapter 6, I apply the principles of procreative permissibility to a very wide variety of cases. I discuss the permissibility of procreating under various natural risk conditions such as genetic diseases, genetic predispositions to physical and mental illness, genetic links to disability, parental age, parental disease, parental disability, and parental (physical) incompetence. In each case, I consider whether it would be rational, under any reasonable conception of rational risk, to accept the risk under consideration as a condition of your own birth in exchange for the freedom to procreate under these risk conditions. Some cases are relatively clear: since Tay-Sachs entails the painful loss of all of one's procreative goods at a very young age with little compensatory or associated benefits, it is a grave and pervasive set of burdens, with a significant probability of occurring if carriers of the Tay-Sachs gene procreate with each other (25%). It is not rational to risk that sort of life for the benefit of being permitted to procreate biologically should you be a Tay-Sachs carrier partnered with another Tay-Sachs carrier. Other cases are more complex, for example, procreation with the risk of achondroplasia or the risk of cognitive disability. Cases can be made either more simple or more complex by the recently available technology known as preimplantation genetic diagnosis (PGD). The availability of PGD can make it easier for us to accept that the 25% risk of cystic fibrosis (CF) that children of coupled carriers of the CF gene run is an irrational risk to accept for the benefit of being morally permitted to procreate if you are one of a coupled carrier of CF. Instead, coupled carriers of CF can use PGD to avoid procreating children with CF. I argue that biological procreation among coupled carriers of CF is impermissible whether PGD is available or not, but the fact that coupled carriers of CF can use PGD to eliminate the risk of CF in their offspring makes it easier to accept what Procreative Balance tells us in this case. In cases of the risk of one discrete physical disability, procreative permissibility will usually permit procreation since it is not irrational to risk having one discrete physical disability in exchange for the freedom to procreate should your children be at risk of one discrete physical disability. This risk assessment is based on the fact that one discrete physical disability will often have limited impact on one's procreative goods or overall well-being, but not being permitted to procreate can have a pervasive effect on one's well-being.

I argue that when there is more than one rational approach to the risk under consideration, we err on the side of permissibility. This is consistent with a pluralistic conception of human good and epistemic humility.

I also apply the principles of procreative permissibility to social procreative risks, such as single parenthood, poverty, and oppression. This is a very complex set of issues, particularly since in the case of poverty or oppression, it can seem unduly harsh to restrict procreativity among people who are otherwise suffering so terribly. On the other hand, it is usually irrational to accept a very significant risk of severe oppression in exchange for the freedom to birth your own children into seriously oppressive conditions. Single parenthood and poverty are hard to tease apart, which can make it difficult to assess them as separate risks. But that is at least in part because being a single parent puts both the parent and the child at a much higher risk for poverty. That alone argues against single parenthood in many (though not all) cases. Poverty, especially severe poverty, like oppression, can present us with a tragic choice: either allow children to be born into abject poverty or remove perhaps the one remaining avenue for human flourishing from those suffering abject poverty. I argue that, despite the tragic nature of this decision, it is irrational to accept a very significant risk of abject poverty in exchange for the freedom to procreate in conditions of abject poverty.

Finally, I apply the principles of procreative permissibility to reproductive technologies, including, in vitro fertilization (IVF), intracytoplasmic sperm injection (ICSI), PGD, savior siblings, gamete donation/sale, and surrogacy. I argue that the problem with experimental reproductive technologies is that they are experimental and, as such, involve experimenting on human subjects without consent. Although parents can give consent to experimentation on behalf of their children, in procreative cases the parents are consenting to further their own procreative interests rather than, as is the case with live sick children, for the sake of the child's own health. This makes parental consent to reproductive technologies a matter of a conflict of interests.

Once reproductive technologies are no longer experimental, we assess the risks they pose just as we assess other sorts of procreative risks. PGD is discussed in detail, and I argue for an intuitive conclusion: PGD is permissible to avoid disease but not to select in favor of disability or for specific traits not associated with health or disease, for example, sex, hair color, or athletic ability. This conclusion is common, but it can be hard to find consistent reasons for this position. I argue that we may distinguish between PGD done for the sake of the child and PGD done for the sake of parental preferences for particular traits. Tailoring your child to have traits you prefer demonstrates that you are not treating your child as an end in herself, a demand implied by the Motivation Restriction. Yet some traits, such as, say, light skin color or male gender, are not selected for to avoid disease or disability yet may be selected by parents for the sake of protecting their children from prejudice, which is done for the child's sake. However, this sort of trait selection is still impermissible for three reasons: First, selecting for skin color or gender is racist or sexist (respectively) and, insofar as it involves participating in prejudice, is wrong for the same reasons it's wrong to be racist or sexist. Second, selecting for traits not associated with disease or disability involves an incorrect conception of human well-being: although there are specific advantages associated with specific traits, such as athletic or musical ability, people with those traits are no more likely to be capable of living a life of human flourishing and achieving human well-being than those who don't have those specific traits. Third, selecting for particular traits is too controlling and, as such, is bad for both parents and children. Exceptions include cases in which a child born with a particular trait would be subject to severe oppression. Savior siblings are discussed at length as well, and gamete donation and surrogacy are also addressed. I argue that gamete donation involves abdication of parental responsibility and, as such, violates the Motivation Restriction and is therefore impermissible. Surrogacy that does not involve gamete donation may sometimes be permissible. Savior siblings are sometimes permissible, depending on whether creating them violates the Motivation Restriction.

A NOTE ON ABORTION

I do not discuss the morality of abortion in this book. The morality of abortion is about who (or what) you can kill. What I am interested in here is questions regarding whom you can create. Once you exist, I can't help you. But there is hope yet for the children you may or may not have. Most of us have children relatively thoughtlessly. Many of us have children we have no moral right to have. Many of us have parents who should not have created us. But many of us have a strong interest in having children, and sometimes it may be permissible. This book will explain how, when, and why procreation may be permissible (or not).

SUGGESTIONS FOR HOW TO READ THIS BOOK

From cover to cover. At least twice. And then a third time with musical and alcoholic accompaniment. If your interests are more specific, however, feel free to read the parts that interest you. Each chapter is readable on its own even though together they form a fairly comprehensive theory of procreative ethics. If you are interested in puzzles regarding what kind of act procreation is and why we might be permissibly motivated to do it, read Chapter 1. If you are interested in a theory of what makes someone parentally responsible (or not), read Chapter 2. If you are interested in the non-identity problem, read Chapter 3. If you are interested in the antinatalist view, read Chapter 4. If you are interested in a theory of procreative permissibility, read Chapter 5. If you would like to see how the theory presented in Chapter 5 applies to real-life cases, read Chapter 6. You should be able to pick and choose what interests you and read accordingly. However, if you are interested in a fairly comprehensive theory of procreative ethics or wonder whether you might be or ought to be so interested, read the whole book.

Chapter 1

Imposing Existence

(A Weighty and Enigmatic Title for a Weighty and Enigmatic Topic)

It's not like chicken.

I'm not sure what we are doing when we decide to create another person, but it's not like chicken. It happens all the time and is as commonplace, sure, but we don't create another person just like chickens create another chicken. We are not a cat among cats or a tree among trees,[1] just part of the world doing its thing. For better or worse, we are conscious, reflective, somewhat rational beings who not only inhabit the world but also try to make some kind of sense of it as well as our place in it. This is not to deny that people, like chickens, are often driven by strong biological or psychological impulses to procreate (nor is it to deny that consciousness or reflection may be a physical process). It is, however, to be skeptical about the claim that pure Darwinian "perpetuation of our genes" behavior is all that is going on when people decide to procreate. This skepticism is supported by the fact that many people seem to curtail their procreativity voluntarily and by the fact that many people who cannot procreate biologically often go to very

---

1. Albert Camus, *The Myth of Sisyphus*, Vintage International, 1991, 51.

great lengths to acquire a child to raise as their own. For as long as people have kept records of themselves, they have told us a bit about how they tried to control when, how, and especially whether, they procreated.[2] Today, contraception is widely available and widely used. It would be difficult, in my view, to maintain that people create as many children as they can successfully raise to reproductive adulthood. Darwinism or the biological instinct to reproduce is unlikely to be anything approximating a complete explanation of human procreativity. It may be possible that, unbeknownst to us, and all appearances notwithstanding, all of our rational explanation and introspection about why we procreate is just silly human chitchat, masking our underlying Darwinian drive. But it seems that the facts of human procreativity argue against that. Of course, biological drive is almost certainly *part* of any complete explanation of human procreativity, but it's not the whole story; it is part of the story. I am interested in the rest of the story. Thus, I will set the purely instinctive or Darwinian explanation aside for now and try to wrap my head around what I take to be one of the most monumental and mystifying things people do: create other people.

It's mind-blowing, really. Here we are, in our strange and vast universe, living with many unknowns, uncertainties, and difficulties, and what do we do? We decide to create a creature like ourselves, a sentient, conscious *person*, with full moral status and a future largely unknown except for the fact that the person will be helpless and dependent for a very long time. How odd of us. Who do we think we are, anyway? Where do we get off? When we procreate, what are we doing and why are we doing it?

---

2. For some intriguing historical references to birth control and abortion techniques, see Will Oremus, "Did Early Christians Practice Birth Control?" *Slate*, February 10, 2012, web (slate.com/articles/news_and_politics/explainer/2012/02/obama_birth_control_battle_when_did_catholics_ban_contraception_.html?wpisrc = slate_river).

In this chapter, I will try to make some sense of procreative actions and motivations. The motivation I am interested in is one that is both explanatory and justifying, meaning, it will accord with the motives that many people actually have when they procreate and it will also be a motive that we find justifiable. I seek a justifiable motive, not necessarily a motive that will, by itself, justify the act. Motivation is morally relevant for its own sake and can also be important to our assessment of an act: it can help justify an act and it can also serve to discredit an act. I don't assume that a justifiable procreative motive will accord with the procreative motives that many people have, but my hope is that it will. I am seeking a justified motive for people's procreative acts to work toward justifying rather than discrediting them (and in order for it to do that work, it has to be a motive that many people have). So that is the kind of motive I'm looking for, and that's why I'm looking for it.

My aim, in so doing, is to make progress toward an understanding of the procreative act so that we can get closer to some kind of legitimate moral peace with it. Procreativity is notoriously riddled with puzzles and paradoxes. I am hoping that if we get a bit more clear on what kind of thing we are doing and what our procreative purposes are, we will be able to clear up some of the puzzles and paradoxes, or at least avoid getting hopelessly entangled in them, and render ourselves more capable of forming a reasonable and action-guiding theory of procreative ethics.

We will want our theory of procreative ethics to enable us to solve or avoid difficult or disturbing procreative puzzles, to be reliably and meaningfully action-guiding in a wide variety of circumstances, to accord with a plausible and palatable account of procreative motivation (one that rings true to the experiences of children and adults), and to be capable of reasonably considering (and likely rejecting) extreme and deeply counterintuitive pro-creative positions, such as procreation is always permissible (even merely as a means of generating organ or labor sources, say) or never permissible (even to great parents in great circum-stances, say).

We have our work cut out for us. As any parent will tell you, procreation is not for the faint of heart.

I   IT'S LIKE ...

What exactly, or even quite roughly, are we doing when we create someone?

(i) A Gift? Those who think that life is fundamentally or intrin-sically good may be sympathetic to the view that life is a gift. If life is a gift, maybe procreation is a generous act of giving the gift of life. But this view, while rosily optimistic, has many confusing and problematic implications. First, if life is a gift, it certainly isn't what anyone always wanted because no one is capable of wanting anything, including life itself, before that person exists. Therefore, unlike some gifts, life itself is neither wanted nor needed by the people to whom it is given.[3] It may be a wonderful "gift" nonethe-less, but, if a gift, it is an atypical one. Moreover, no matter how good life can be, it can be terrible at times, and it can sometimes be pretty bad, beginning to bitter end, even by the most optimistic

---

3. At least not in advance. People may want to keep their life once they have it but that is not the same thing as wanting or needing it before or when it is "given" to them. This differs from the claim that we cannot give the gift of life because there is no one to give it to. It is not conceptually impossible to think of creating a gift and its recipient simultaneously (I owe this idea to David Velleman). I discuss a variant of this claim in subsection IV (i) "Imposing Existence."

accounts, so it is often literally one hell of a gift. (Skeptical? Consider your odds of a life from hell if you are born a girl today in Afghanistan or Saudi Arabia, born African American in the United States in 1830, born a Jew in Europe in the Middle Ages or 1935, etc. Not only can this list be long, it includes large numbers of people and many time periods.) And even the very best life is, unlike most gifts, a *job*. It demands our hard work and attention. If I give you a violin, you may have to work at enjoying it, especially if you don't know how to play it; if I give you a book, it may take some engagement on your part to enjoy it. Some gifts require work to be enjoyed, but most gifts won't harm you if you do nothing with them. The book can sit there unread, be regifted, or tossed out. The violin can be ignored. Not so life. If you don't work at it, you will likely suffer. It is hard to conceive of a good life that doesn't take any work to build or maintain. The building and maintaining of a good life may be the very thing that makes it good, but that still makes it difficult to think of life as a gift. A gift comes free (or at least ignorable); a good life does not. For these reasons, I find gift giving an ill-fitting analogy for procreativity.

(ii) A Predicament? Considering the work (and luck) it takes to achieve a good life, David Velleman argues that procreation is like putting someone in a "predicament;" people are born needing to make a good life for themselves and will likely suffer greatly if they fail.[4] The fact that people are born helpless and need to be nurtured effectively in order to have a reasonable shot at overcoming their predicament and achieving human well-being is reason, Velleman argues, to hold parents particularly responsible to nurture them, just as if you plan to throw a kid into a pool,

---

4. David Velleman, "The Gift of Life," *Philosophy and Public Affairs* 2008 36: 245–266.

you should teach her how to swim and rescue her if she seems to be drowning.[5] But the pool analogy does not reflect very well on the ones doing the throwing because we generally do not think of putting people into predicaments as a morally laudable thing to do. If procreation is really like putting people into predicaments, we probably should stop doing that. Predicament: def. "**difficult situation**, a difficult, unpleasant, or embarrassing situation from which there is no clear or easy way out."[6] Sounds like life to me, but it doesn't sound like what people think they are doing when they decide to have a baby (it's not among the commonly discussed or recognized procreative aims).[7] If that's what procreators do, why do they do it?

(iii) A (Worthwhile) Risk? Because swimming is fun and worth the risk, presumably. There is a risk of drowning, but the risk is not great and can be greatly mitigated by careful and informed practices.[8] So maybe procreation is like imposing a risk, which can perhaps be justified if the risk is worth taking and is imposed on future people for their own good or at least not contrary to their good. Thinking of procreation as a risk imposition may serve as a middle ground between the dreamily unrealistic "gifting" analogy and the perplexing and damning "predicament putting" analogy. It tells us that procreation may be justified when the risk has a good chance of ripening into a good and avoiding a negative outcome, or something along these lines.

---

5. Velleman, "The Gift of Life."
6. *Encarta* Dictionary (web).
7. This is not an empirical claim. It is a kind of common-sense view.
8. Whether the risk can be mitigated by the suicide option that is open to most people is debatable. I discuss this question in Chapter 4, along with questions regarding subjective perceptions of well-being.

But it still leaves us wondering why we do it (remember that the motive we seek is one that is both explanatory and justifiable). If procreation is a case of risk imposition, in order to evaluate the morality of the risk imposition we will want to know more about why we are doing it because whether it's morally permissible to impose a risk on others depends, in part, on why we are imposing the risk. Is it vital to our projects? Is it something that we are confident the person upon whom we are imposing the risk would want us to do? Are we doing it to benefit them? Getting clear on our motives for imposing the risks of life on our children may help us assess the morality of the risk imposition.

It is not entirely clear why we would go to the trouble of imposing a (worthwhile, presumably) risk on a future person and it is notoriously puzzling to consider whether we can reasonably claim to be doing so for the future person's own good. After all, the future person does not have a good or any state at all to improve, benefit, or better until after the procreative act is complete. When we think about why we procreate, does it ring true to say, "Life is so great that I wanted to impose it on someone for her own good"? That is not an answer I often—or, more accurately, ever—hear; and I often ask the question. Generally speaking, when we impose risks on others, we do so for our own sake and justify it by the nature of the risk, the likelihood of it ripening into a harm, the cost to us of not imposing it, and the cost to others of our imposing it upon them. However, we also often impose risks on children for their own good, for example, when we teach them how to swim or ride a bicycle.[9] Still, it does seem odd to cite children's own good to explain why we impose all of life's risks upon them and it also does not seem to accord

---

9. I discuss the implications of this further in Chapter 4.

with the reasons people say that they choose to procreate (i.e., the reason is not explanatory). Moreover, if life is a risk, it is not altogether clear that it is a worthwhile risk to take or impose (i.e., the reason may not be justifiable). Not only are there many ways for life to turn out really badly, there is also the matter of how wildly and incredibly uncertain life is. Adults who have been screened for all screenable genetic diseases may still give birth to a severely deformed, ill, disabled, suffering person; adults well placed to care for a child can drop dead anytime, lose their jobs, blow up their heretofore stable relationships; prosperous, productive societies can degenerate into civil war, anarchy, tyranny, and oppression; anyone can get what we might call a great start in life and come to a horrific end (and middle). Is it prudent to place a bet with stakes so high and outcomes almost unfathomably uncertain? Is it permissible? We would at least have to have a very good reason. And so we return to the question of why we procreate.

If we are going to impose so tricky a risk on another person and if we care to justify the imposition, it seems that examining our motivations may be an important place to start. If our motives can be genuinely related to the child's own good or at least not contrary to the child's good, that might provide us with a promising place from which to consider the rest of the procreative moral picture. Some might think that this will not be that difficult.

II PROCREATIVE MOTIVATION IS OBVIOUS AND NOT PROBLEMATIC (?)

(i) For the Child It might seem obvious to some that procreation is done for our children because raising children usually

involves significant sacrifice for their sake. "At four in the morning when I am soothing an upset child or cleaning up his vomit, a child who has been doing the four a.m. thing for four weeks in a row, ask me about for whose sake I procreated," one might say. Parenting with any degree of adequacy demands sacrifice and generosity, but this fact does not automatically provide us with a procreative motive that both accords with our experiences and seems justifiable. Creating a person and raising a person, while related, are not the same activity. Just because raising children involves sacrificing for their sake that does not mean that creating children is an act of sacrifice for their sake. Claiming to procreate for the sake of the child is similar to viewing life as a gift bestowed on the child and is problematic for the same reasons.

(ii) Adding Value to the World If we think that people are valuable or if we think that the loving parent-child relationship is valuable, it may seem obvious that we procreate to add value to the world. Put less additively, we may think that people are awe-inspiring and that procreation is a way to create something of extraordinary value.[10] Perhaps. However, there are some difficulties with this happy approach to procreative motivation. First, even if it would be a motive that we find justifiable, it is less than explanatory. Most people do not procreate in order to add awe-inspiring value, or even just plain old value, to the world. It is a highly intellectual and impersonal way of conceiving of procreation and it requires a rather removed and rare view about value, people, and

10. I thank my happy and awe-inspiring friends Paul Hurley and Saul Smilansky for raising these points. See also Smilansky, "Is There a Moral Obligation to Have Children?" *Journal of Applied Philosophy* 1995 12: 41–53.

the world. I do not think the value-added procreative motivation accords with experience.[11]

And lucky it doesn't because it is not as justifiable as it might initially seem. First, as a way of adding value to the world, it is a very risky and high-handed way. Some people, such as country music singers or, if you must, Hitler, detract value from the world. Many other people, while very valuable, suffer greatly and it may not seem right to have procreated them to add value to the world despite their great suffering. Some theologians have tried to explain why some babies are born very sick or why good people wind up extremely disabled for long periods of time by saying that these babies or sick people provide us with an opportunity to be caring and giving. But it would not be respectful of people to create them as sources of do-gooding for others. Similarly, it seems problematic to claim to create people as sources of value when those people are at risk of great suffering. There are other ways to add value to the world that don't involve these risks. We can enhance the relationships we already have or develop new relationships with existing people in order to add the value of loving relationships to the world. We can create works of art or help existing people in order to create things of value or express how valuable and awe inspiring people are. It might seem better to create or enhance value in these more reliable ways than to procreate.

Further difficulties with the value-added procreative motivation are that it makes procreation seem cold and impersonal, almost like we are treating the future person or our loving relationship with that person as a piece of value to add to the stack of

11. Similarly, the idea that we might procreate because, from a cosmic standpoint, life is cool, rare, and valuable is not explanatory—it is not the reason that most people (even David Enoch, who suggested this reason to me) have children.

value in the world. Imagining your parents deciding to create you to add value to the world can seem rather distant and lonely. Imagining your parents deciding to create you to add another loving relationship to the world can seem similarly distant and uncozy. These reasons have nothing to do with *you* or even with your parents. They are about an abstract value or about the *world* (Who is that? Do we like her?).

Finding a procreative motive that accords with experience and is morally justifiable is neither obvious nor unproblematic. As crazy as it might seem to desperately sacrificing middle-of-the-night parents in awe of the beautiful and valuable babies they are sacrificing for, it will not be easy to find procreative motives that don't make procreators look . . . well, *bad*.

A look at some of the puzzling aspects of procreation can serve to highlight some of our problematic procreative motives. I turn now to those puzzles. I begin with puzzles about procreative motivation and then proceed to more metaphysical procreative puzzles.

III   PROCREATIVE MOTIVE PUZZLES:
A SAMPLING

(i) Autonomy We[12] love autonomy (especially our own). We value being moral agents, making our own choices, running our own lives, creating our own meaning, and choosing our own projects.[13] For many, it is not only a great good but also the

---

12. The "we" in this section refers to contemporary liberal and pseudoliberal societies and peo-ple. Not all people, but lots and lots of them (especially since I'm talking about individuals and not about governments, states, or societies).

13. See Bernard Williams, "A Critique of Utilitarianism," *Utilitarianism For and Against*, J. J. C. Smart and Bernard Williams, Cambridge University Press, 1973 and Robert Nozick, *Anarchy, State, and Utopia*, Basic Books, 1974, 45–51.

highest or most important good. Autonomy is a fundamental value for both Kantian ethics and liberal society. For those less intoxicated by autonomy, it is usually still considered an important value that we seek for ourselves and try to respect in others. Thus, we procreate intending to try to raise our children to be capable of autonomy and, ultimately, to be autonomous.[14] Yet we create them entirely without their permission or consent. Since future people are not capable of consenting to anything, some may find it unproblematic that we create them without their consent. Some may even consider worrying about future persons' consent to having been procreated to be a category mistake, akin to wondering whether the color red is even or odd.[15] But we can agree that a future person is not the kind of thing that can consent and yet view that as a way of *describing* the discomfort we feel about forcing the person into existence rather than a way of alleviating it. Others go further, and argue that the fact that we can't obtain future persons' consent to being procreated makes all procreation seriously morally problematic.[16] We need not settle this now[17] because we can agree that we cannot ask future people if they'd wish to accept an invitation to the existence party and note that, to whatever extent this is problematic, we certainly can seek other relationships and activities that are not problematic in

---

14. See Joel Feinberg regarding our responsibilities to safeguard our children's future autonomy rights so that they can meaningfully exercise them as adults. He calls this the child's "right to an open future": "The Child's Right to an Open Future," in *Whose Child? Children's Rights, Parental Authority, and State Power*, William Aiken and Hugh Lafollette, Eds., Littlefield, Adams, 1980, 125–153.
15. I thank Charles Young for this point.
16. Seana Shiffrin, "Wrongful Life, Procreative Responsibility, and the Significance of Harm," *Legal Theory* 1999 5: 117–148. Shiffrin's autonomy-based challenge to the moral legitimacy of procreative ethics has been extremely influential.
17. I discuss this issue in Chapter 4.

this way. Therefore, procreation can seem unduly coercive. Why do we want to act that way? It seems contrary to our reflectively endorsed values. Puzzling.

(ii) Equality We value equality and we wish to be treated as equals in most of our relationships.[18] If we are morally admirable people, we try to treat others that way as well. A relationship of equals is consistent with our value of autonomy and, in that way, seems laudable and respectful. So why do we deliberately seek to procreate and thereby enter into a hopelessly unequal relationship, and one with the balance of power tipped entirely in our own direction? Not only is the parent-child relationship unequal, it is predictably unequal for a very long time and, arguably, for the most important part of the relationship and for the time for which many seek it out. Thinking of procreation in this way can make it seem manipulative, like we are creating an incompetent person so that we can have the sort of unequal relationship that we may value. Of course, many admirable relationships are clearly unequal, involving a competent benefactor and a less competent beneficiary.[19] This sort of inequality is not necessarily problematic when it occurs naturally—that is, when the beneficiary of our paternalism exists already and needs our help—but it can seem less savory when we are creating a person in a needy state deliberately because we want the care-taking relationship. Again we arrive at an embarrassing motive that seems contrary to our reflectively endorsed values.

18. Of course, some of our relationships are unequal in some respects, as in an employee/supervisor relationship, but those relationships are entered into voluntarily and for mutual benefit, and they are also limited to one aspect of our lives. If they define or completely pervade our lives, they are likely to be thought of as objectionably unequal.

19. Some view their relationships with their pets this way, but it would be disrespectful to treat a person as a pet. (I'm not so thrilled with the unequal human-pet relationships that exemplify this either but I don't expect a lot of agreement there . . .)

(iii) Benevolence We try to be kind. We value benevolence and try to practice it. We want to express our capacity for love and beneficence. But although we have many opportunities to be loving and benevolent toward people who exist already in a variety of ways and in different kinds of relationships and capacities, we choose to devote a good deal (and often nearly all) of our capacity for love and benevolence toward beings seemingly created for that very purpose—to be the subjects of our love and benevolence. If we take a step back and note that procreation involves the deliberate creation of persons in desperate need of our care, love, and benevolence, procreation can smack of manipulation and disrespect to the persons deliberately created to be the recipients of that care, love, and benevolence. ("I created you because I wanted someone to take care of and be loving to," we might imagine a benevolent parent saying. "Thanks a lot," whimpers the utterly helpless, needy baby. "Glad I could help you out.")

(iv) Altruism We value giving to others and we disapprove of undue selfishness. We especially disapprove of the kind of selfishness that involves not only undue regard for oneself but also insufficient regard for others. People often say that they want to have children so that they can grow beyond their selfish concerns and personal desires. They want to be less selfish and more giving. Having children is often seen as a way to achieve or express these admirable goals, and choosing not to have children is often seen as selfish.[20] Yet when prospective parents talk about giving as a reason to have children, they are talking about themselves and becoming the people that they want to become. Children can seem

---

20. Joe O'Connor, "Trend of Couples Not Having Children Is Just Plain Selfish," *National Post*, September 19, 2012; Briana Mowry, "Is Being Childfree by Choice Selfish?" *Redbook Magazine*, web (redbookmag.com/love-sex/advice/childfree-by-choice); among many others.

like a mere means to parental ends of personal growth because the prospective parents are referring to their own ends, goals, and desires only. This too can make parental motives seem manipulative, disrespectful, and even selfish (yes, *selfish* in procreating even though *raising* children demands sacrifice and devotion to another—that's part of the puzzle).

This only adds to the very long list of traditional and common reasons for procreating that can easily sound selfish, involving insufficient regard for those affected by one's actions: having children to work one's farm, to take care of oneself in one's old age, to satisfy social expectations, to carry on the family name, to secure a sense of immortality,[21] and so on.

This is disheartening. It appears far too easy to characterize our procreative motives as arrogant, manipulative, coercive, selfish, reckless, and hubristic. Not only does this way of thinking about procreation make most adults seem guilty of serious moral crimes, it also does not fit with the way that most people think of procreation. Procreation is often thought of as good, generous, the way to end a comedy and live a rich and full life. Moreover, this way of thinking about procreation is common from the perspective of both adults and children, most of whom don't see their very existence as a wrong perpetrated upon them by their parents.[22] So what is missing from our list of procreative

---

21. Carrying on the family name and securing a sense of immortality can be other-regarding reasons for procreating if it is done not from personal concerns or interests but for the benefit of one's ancestors who may have had these interests and are, arguably, partly dependent on descendants to further them. I thank Yuval Avnur for this point.

22. There are notable and voluble exceptions. I myself am partial to this exceptional view—I feel victimized to have been brought into existence, and I feel guilty for having brought my own children into existence, but I realize that this is a very uncommon way to see the world. Though not entirely unique, of course. See David Benatar, *Better Never to Have Been: The Harm of Coming into Existence*, Oxford University Press, 2006.

motivations? Which motive is going to be less puzzling, less paradoxical, less morally objectionable, and more consistent with everyday experiences and perspectives? I will return to this question in section V.

IV   PROCREATIVE METAPHYSICAL PUZZLES? NO. IT'S THE MORAL PROBLEM, STUPID

If we knew what we were doing, maybe we would have a better idea of why we do it. It can be hard to understand why we are doing something when we are not clear on what that something is. Therefore, in an effort to understand procreative motivation, it might help us to get clearer on what procreation is. But when we try to do that, we seem to run into metaphysical puzzles. Procreation is not so easy to understand. Metaphysically, it may look like procreation is a special and difficult case, an inherently confusing case where it is especially difficult to figure out what, metaphysically, is going on. And it then seems reasonable to think that we must find a way to resolve our metaphysics in order to address procreative moral issues. This, however, is false. The metaphysical mysteries are either solved relatively easily or can be left unresolved without undue moral anxiety—they are not morally pressing.

(i) Imposing Existence   It seems that procreation is something that existing people do to nonexistent people, but there are no people who don't exist and, even if there were, how could we interact with or do anything to the nonexistent? So whom are we procreating? It's confusing. People come with existence already firmly in place—it's not as if we conceive babies and then

pierce their ears and dress them in existence; all babies are existent. We may give our children puppies and blankets, but not existence. Another way to express this worry is that if existence is not a property, we cannot give it to anyone. This makes it incongruous to speak, as many often do, of "bringing someone into existence," imposing existence on future people, or giving existence (or even life) to one's children. Yet it does feel like we are imposing, causing, or giving existence when we procreate; it's part of the way we think of procreative acts, yet it is not easy to express this natural way of thinking without running into confusion and controversy over using existence as a predicate or property.[23]

I suggest we think of what goes on when we, say, take paint and canvas and create a painting, a beautiful (or hideous) work of art. Have we "imposed" existence upon the painting? Hardly. We created the painting and we may be the most relevant cause of its existence, but it wasn't there to be imposed upon and it does not seem all that metaphysically problematic to take paint, canvas, and brush and, by putting them together in various ways, create a painting. In the same way, we take gametes and put them together, and they grow into a person. It may be biologically fascinating and metaphysically mysterious in the sense in which everything is (what exists? why does anything exist? what does it mean to exist? what does it mean to take from existing things and make a new thing? what counts as new? what counts as things?), but it is not mysterious in a way that is particular to procreation. What makes it more intuitive to think of imposing existence on a person than

---

23. Whether "existence" is a property attributable to entities is a long-standing debate in metaphysics. See entry on "Existence" in *The Stanford Encyclopedia of Philosophy* (web) for a synopsis of the history of this debate.

on a painting is that a person is capable of experience, reflection, consent, autonomy, and opinions. A person can object to having been created; a person can have an opinion about her very existence. A painting has no experiences and is certainly not capable of or entitled to autonomy or the kind of moral consideration to which persons are entitled. It's not like anything to be a painting. That's why we worry much less about creating a painting[24] than creating a person. But the procreative worry, to whatever extent we do or should have this worry, is moral, not metaphysical. We don't worry about whether we have been just, benevolent, manipulative, or coercive to the painting because the painting is not, on most views, a moral subject. This illustrates that, for our purposes, metaphysically, we create persons much as we create paintings. It's the morality of our procreativity that's special (in that it involves causing persons to exist, which is morally complicated and precarious), not its metaphysics.

(ii) The Non-Identity Problem It is difficult, when procreating, to identify the person harmed by acts that seem to be clear cases of reprehensible procreative negligence. It seems implausible to say that whichever child is conceived in these cases has been harmed. To use Parfit's famous example, if a fourteen-year-old girl decides to have a baby, can we use reasons of the future child's good to persuade her to wait until she is more mature and more capable of taking care of a baby? Intuitively, the answer is clearly yes, because having a teen mother usually poses significant difficulties for the child. But which child? We don't seem to be able to identify any child for whom the mother's act is worse than her alternatives

---

24. Creating a painting does have its own set of worries, including aesthetic worries and possibly even moral worries, depending on the view one has about creative responsibility and art.

because, for any child the fourteen-year-old might now conceive, so long as the child's life is likely to be worth living, despite its difficult origins, it is not bad for the child to exist, and if the fourteen-year-old girl had waited until she was twenty-five to procreate, she would have created a different child (made from gametes released at a later date and with a different genetic and environmental profile). This problem applies at the level of population policy as well because all policies affect timelines and time affects which sperm will fertilize which egg, thereby affecting identity. To avoid sanctioning these types of procreative negligence, a theory of procreative ethics will either have to solve or avoid the non-identity problem.

The non-identity problem can be described as a metaphysical surprise: the person you thought you were harming by what you took to be your procreative negligence of teen motherhood actually turns out to be the person not so harmed since her life is worth living and she would not exist had you acted with a more appropriate degree of procreative care. You trash the environment, which you think will harm future people. But, surprise! The people who will suffer from the trashed environment wouldn't have existed if you hadn't trashed it (because trashing the environment affects when and with whom people procreate and, therefore, is itself an identity-determining act or policy), so, by metaphysical sleight of hand, you trashed the environment but harmed no one.[25] This

---

25. Melinda Roberts argues that in some non-identity cases, there is a tiny but not nonexistent possibility that some individuals would exist whether the act in question, such as the trashing of the environment, occurs or not. See Roberts, *Child versus Childmaker*, Rowman & Littlefield, 1998. Others argue for distinguishing certain kinds of non-identity cases from others, e.g., Hanser distinguishes between parents and policymakers (Matthew Hanser, "Harming Future People," *Philosophy and Public Affairs* 1990 19: 47–70). Usually dividing non-identity cases into different categories is done when someone has a solution for cases in one category but not another. Since I will solve the non-identity problem for all cases (in Chapter 3), I will not discuss the different ways one might divvy them up.

is indeed a metaphysical surprise, but it could remain a harmless or even charming curiosity if it didn't generate what many take to be a moral problem. We think that procreating at fourteen or trashing the environment is straightforwardly morally wrong or, at best, suboptimal, because it is usually very difficult to grow up with a teen mother and it is tough to grow up in a trashed environment. Creating these adverse conditions (without a justifying reason or excuse) seems harmful and wrong. The fact that the non-identity problem makes it hard for us to justify these strong moral intuitions is a moral problem. It may have a metaphysical solution, though it is more commonly solved or avoided morally, but it is only a problem because it creates a moral problem. If it did not create a moral problem, we could easily live with non-identity as a metaphysical surprise or curiosity. It is the moral problem of non-identity that demands our attention, not the metaphysical one. If we could only solve the moral problem by solving the metaphysical problem, then we would have to attend to the metaphysical problem, but our attention to the metaphysical problem would be derivative, derived from our unwillingness to accept its moral implications. As it turns out, most suggested solutions to the non-identity problem are moral, not metaphysical.[26]

---

26. There are way too many moral solutions to list, but here are a few favorites: Paul Hurley and Rivka Weinberg, "Whose Problem Is Non-identity?," *Journal of Moral Philosophy*, forthcoming; James Woodward, "The Non-identity Problem," *Ethics* 1986 96: 805–831; Matthew Hanser, "Harming Future People," *Philosophy and Public Affairs* 1990 19: 47–70; David Velleman, "Love and Nonexistence," *Philosophy and Public Affairs* 2008 36: 266–288; David Wasserman, "The Non-identity Problem, Disability, and the Role Morality of Prospective Parents," *Ethics* 2005 116: 132–152; and Gregory Kavka, "The Paradox of Future Individuals," *Philosophy and Public Affairs* 1981 11: 93–112. For a metaphysical solution to the non-identity problem, see Rivka Weinberg, "Identifying and Dissolving the Non-identity Problem," *Philosophical Studies* 2008 137: 3–18.

And see Chapter 3.

However, even if none of the proposed solutions works to solve the non-identity problem, the problem can be avoided by some central moral theories because the problem is aimed at moral theories that determine wrongdoing based on how an act affects specific, identifiable individuals,[27] that is, narrow person-affecting theories. Neither consequentialism nor contractualism is a *narrow* person-affecting theory.[28] Consequentialism is not person-affecting at all; that is, it does not assess the morality of an action based on its effect on persons. Instead, consequentialism looks at how actions affect the resulting states of affairs. Therefore, most consequentialists think that consequentialism avoids the non-identity problem.[29] Contractualism looks at how actions affect people regardless of identity—it is a *wide* person-affecting theory—and, therefore, can also be taken to avoid the non-identity problem.[30] Virtue ethics focuses on the cultivation and expression of character traits and is therefore unaffected by a problem aimed at theories that can only call an action wrong if it harms a specific person. Thus, the metaphysical problem of non-identity will pose a moral problem only if we reject all of the many proposed solutions and also reject the avoidance of the problem claimed by some central moral theories, and also feel that non-identity is a metaphysical puzzle that cannot be set aside unsolved. That set of views seems somewhat extreme to me and in need of its own defense. For our purposes, it seems reasonable to set the non-identity problem aside for now. (I'll solve it later.)[31]

---

27. This is, arguably, an advantage those theories have for purposes of procreative ethics.
28. I refer here to classic versions of act or rule consequentialism.
29. This claim has been disputed. See Hurley and Weinberg, "Whose Problem Is Non-identity?"
30. See Rivka Weinberg, "Procreative Justice: A Contractualist Account," *Public Affairs Quarterly* 2002 16: 405–425.
31. I will address the non-identity problem and its implications at length in Chapter 3.

(iii) The Hotel California Is existence, like the Hotel California,[32] inescapable? One might think that death is tantamount to or results in nonexistence. Yet it may not be so easy to wipe the slate clean of yourself, so to speak, because, even after death, you exist as a subject of reference, as a legal entity with power to distribute your assets in accordance with the wishes you had while alive, in the memory of others, and as a physical presence in the world (if you are buried, your molecules join the world's eventually; if you are cremated, same goes for your ashes, etc.).[33] There is a reason our bones, dust, or ash is referred to as "remains;" it *remains*. If existence is irrevocable, procreation is an even greater imposition on those not asked whether they wish to exist because they are stuck with what we did to them forever. Perhaps not stuck in any significant or relevant way but, still, it seems to me that we might be less than fully comfortable with imposing something so weighty, risky, and *permanent* on another person.

Existence may be inescapable, but that, by itself, poses no special moral difficulty because we seem to cease to exist as subjects of experience after we die. We are familiar with the law of conservation of matter; we understand that our atoms will persist after we disintegrate, but we have no reason to care very much about that. We may think that once we cease to exist as moral agents, upon our deaths, we cease to exist in any sense we care about, so

---

32. Famous Eagles song, 1977. As the song implies, the kind of inescapability I'm talking about is the colloquial sense of inescapability. I'm not talking about metaphysical neccesity.

33. This differs from the ontological status of, say, the tooth fairy or a round square. Dead people are neither fictional nor impossible. They are dead but whether that is exactly the same as nonexistent is not clear. See Fred Feldman, *Confrontations with the Reaper*, Oxford University Press, 1992 and Daniel Sperling, *Posthumous Interests*, Cambridge University Press, 2008.

who cares if our atoms, once dearranged from what was us, rearrange and join with others to become tulips? As people, unless there is an afterlife, we eventually cease to exist as subjects of experience. Whether we persist as moral subjects anyway, with posthumous interests, is the subject of ongoing debate,[34] but it is hard to imagine that our interests persist forever. However, if one does think that the interests of persons persist forever, the reason to care about this is a moral reason. We may want to understand the nature and extent of our responsibilities both to dead people and to the people we choose to create, especially since their interests will be permanent (on this view). Here too, it is the morality that is salient, not the metaphysics, and it does not look like we have much of a moral problem. (The only cases that may present a moral problem are cases of permanent posthumous interests, and it is difficult to support the claim that those sorts of interests exist. We can therefore leave the moral problem to those who maintain that dead people have permanent persistent interests.)

We may stop worrying about metaphysics. Our serious procreative worries are moral.

V WE'RE IN THIS TOGETHER? PROCREATING AS FORMING A PARENT-CHILD RELATIONSHIP

I now return to the question left open at the end of section III, namely, is there a procreative motive that we can truly understand, embrace, connect with, and deem justifiable? A motive that is both explanatory and justified? I suggest that the desire to engage in the

34. See, for example, Sperling, *Posthumous Interests.*

parent-child relationship as a parent and to participate in a family may be a procreative motive that we can both make sense of and reflectively endorse.[35] Let's call this the *parental motive* and investigate some notable aspects of its nature.

(i) A Unique Relationship Being a parent is life structuring and life altering. It has a deep and pervasive impact on one's life and can be seen as a symbiotic relationship with one's children in the context of family life.[36] The parent-child relationship, ideally, is mutually beneficial and respectful. That is not to say that it is beneficial to the child to have been created but, rather, that it is beneficial to the child, once it exists, to participate in a nurturing and respectful parent-child relationship. To procreate motivated by the desire to participate in this kind of a relationship seems reasonably respectful and understandable. The parent-child relationship affords the parties to the relationship goods that are both unique and valuable, and, therefore, the desire to engage in parenting and participate in this way in a unique familial relationship is not a desire that can readily be met in other ways. It's not as if one can be nice to kittens or volunteer as a mentor for a disadvantaged child and feel like one has been affected in the same way as one can be by engaging fully in parenting one's child. Parenting can be engaged in without demeaning children since it is not inherently demeaning to be cared for as a child. If one is raised with developmentally

---

35. There may, of course, be other motives that have not occurred to me and that might survive reflection; I offer one that has. Christine Overall suggests a related "best reason" to have a child. She argues that the desire to create a new relationship that is particularly meaningful to shaping the identity of both the parent and child is the best reason to procreate. See Overall, *Why Have Children? The Ethical Debate*, MIT Press, 2012, Chapter 10.
36. The life-altering aspect of parenthood occurs with one's first child. It is far less marked with each successive child. I discuss the implications of this fact in Chapter 6.

appropriate respect and autonomy and is encouraged to mature into an autonomous adult, it does not seem that one has been thereby demeaned or used.[37]

(ii) Symbiotic, Respectful, but Not Undertaken to Benefit Children Of course, unlike adults who can choose to engage in parenting and to participate in a family, children have their part in the parent-child relationship thrust upon them and in a way that cannot be said to *benefit* them, without significant controversy. Some philosophers claim that having been created is good for a person; others argue just as strongly that having been created is bad for a person, but few argue that having been created is of *benefit* to a person because, like harm, benefit is usually analyzed counterfactually: you are considered harmed by an act if it makes you worse off than you would have otherwise been and benefited if it makes you better off than you would have otherwise been. Thus, even if the child's life is good for the child once the child exists, it is still not a benefit to the child to have been procreated. That's why we cannot easily claim to create a child to further the child's interests. The child has interests only *if* the child exists; otherwise we have no real subject for interests at all. Therefore we do not further the child's interests by bringing it into existence.[38] We must face the fact that we don't procreate for the sake of our children. We procreate because we want to. Hopefully, we want

---

37. If we created children to keep them as children, forever dependent on us, that could well be seen as demeaning, and as improperly using children, given that children, in the usual case, are capable of growing into autonomous adults. If we select for children who are disabled in ways that will prevent them from reaching autonomous adulthood because we want our nurturing and caregiving roles to persist indefinitely, that too seems an improper use of the child and inconsistent with the way we ought to aspire to treat another person.

38. The phrase "bringing into existence" is somewhat misleading as it can conjure up a picture of taking someone from one place to another when, in fact, procreation involves the creation of a new subject, not facilitating the travel of an existent subject.

to because we want to engage in the parent-child relationship as a parent and participate in a family. Thus we come to an understanding of how we may procreate with a justifiable motive. The parental motive seems justifiable because acting on it may satisfy a unique and legitimate interest of existing people and, arguably, may do so in a way that can be respectful of the future child before the child is conceived and beneficial to the child once the child exists.

This does not assume that everything we do is either for our own sake or for the sake of another; we do things for many reasons, some of which involve ourselves and others, others of which involve things we may value, for example, art, nature, science, regardless of its personal impact on ourselves or other people.[39] I have argued against procreating purely as an expression of objective value on both experiential and moral grounds. We may procreate because we want to engage in the parent-child relationship as a parent and participate in family life. Hopefully, that is usually not objectionably selfish but, rather, respectful of the child.

Since the parental motive is one that seems both plausible and palatable, it might be worth considering what can be good about family life for its participants.

a) *Nurturing and Being Nurtured*: It is good to nurture and be nurtured. Nurturing another person can be gratifying to the parent, and it is comforting and vital to be nurtured as a child. A paradigmatic example of how rewarding a nurturing relationship can be for both parties to it is breastfeeding. Breastfeeding

---

39. For an extended discussion of this view and its implications, see Susan Wolf, *Meaning in Life and Why It Matters*, Princeton University Press, 2010.

is often very rewarding for the parent (it doesn't hurt that it can result in a hormone-induced euphoria), and most babies seem to love it and to find it deeply satisfying. (In fact, one benefit of breastfeeding for the mother is that she can experience how great it can feel to satisfy another person so completely.) As children grow, nurturing and being nurtured can continue to be mutually satisfying though, of course, it becomes more complex and more difficult but, at the same time, richer and more human.[40]

b) *Family Ties*: When our family ties don't gag, unduly constrain, or choke us, they can be a source of great friendship, intimacy, and security. Family loyalty and generosity is usually more reliable and magnanimous than the kind of loyalty and generosity typically experienced in nonfamilial relationships. That's why people who are out of a job or a place to live will more often be found in their parent's home or sister's basement than on their friend's couch (that couch is usually good only for a short-term stay). People can often find joy, guidance, and comfort in the physical, emotional, and temperamental similarities often found within families and can feel alienated, lonely, and adrift in their absence.[41] It's somehow enjoyable when you all laugh the same way, and it can be comforting and instructive to see how your relatives handle the anxiety you have in common. The history of shared experiences is something that is not only often valued but also can be valued more as we age. Family can be a source of deep, reliable, and long-lasting intimacy, love,

---

40. That is not to imply that breastfeeding is anything less than fully human. It's ridiculous to hear people say that the idea of breastfeeding makes them feel like a cow. Why doesn't the cow feel like you? (I owe that insight to Miriam Perr.)

41. See Velleman, "The Gift of Life."

familiarity, comfort, and guidance. That's pretty good, as relationships go, and it can be just as good for parents as it can be for their children, both as children and as the adults into which they grow.[42]

(iii) What Really Happens I'm not saying this is *what happens* when people have children. Family can be suffocating, humiliating, and abusive in ways unmatched by other relationships we might have. Most children who are murdered are murdered by their parents(!)[43] And many people procreate for reasons wholly unrelated to the more respectable ones just discussed. Many people procreate without thinking very much about it at all or entirely "by accident," due to either lack of contraceptive use or contraceptive failure. While there may be no disrespect felt if one is created by thoughtless natural or accidental processes, the way, say, that a plant might grow from seeds blown by the wind into the soil and then rained upon, there may be disrespect felt if moral agents create you without any thought or care about the person you will turn out to be and the life you are likely to lead. Thoughtless procreation, in my view, does display a rather reckless disregard for the magnitude of the effects and implications of creating another person. People are valuable and ought to be treated with consideration—that is elementary and uncontroversial—so it is not much of a stretch to say that thoughtless procreation is morally reckless and, at least in that respect, negligent.

---

42. See Marissa Diener and Mary Beth Diener McGavran, "What Makes People Happy? A Developmental Approach to the Literature on Family Relationships and Well-Being," in *The Science of Subjective Well-Being*, Michael Eid and Randy J. Larson, Eds., Guilford Press, 2008, 347–375.
43. See Timothy Y. Mariano, Heng Choon (Oliver) Chan, and Wade C. Myers, "Toward a More Holistic Understanding of Filicide: A Multidisciplinary Analysis of 32 Years of U.S. Arrest Data," *Forensic Science International* 2014 236: 46–53.

However, there are many procreative cases that might initially seem insufficiently thoughtful or respectful but that are probably, on closer inspection, more similar to the parental motive than might otherwise appear. It is not uncommon for people to say that they had children because it seemed like "the next step" either in their lives or in their relationships. That can sound very selfish or thoughtless (who wants to think that her very existence was predicated on nothing more than her being "the next step"?). But that depends on where one is walking. The "next step" in a rich, full, and rewarding life, once one becomes a stable adult, may be becoming a parent. Similarly, the "next step" in a loving, stable relationship may be to expand into a family by engaging in parenting. The parental motive may be implied in the seemingly bland, rote "next step" reason for procreating. It is also not uncommon for people to say that they had children because they "just wanted to" or they "always wanted to" or even because "kids are cute" or "I've always loved kids." These reasons can sound thoughtless or selfish, but more charitably, and I would guess more accurately, interpreted, they too are ways of expressing a desire to engage in parenting; they too may often be instances of the parental procreative motivation (though they still bespeak a need for more serious and explicit moral reflection). They may not be instances of the parental procreative motivation, which would be unfortunate, and I have no way to establish firmly that they must be, but my interpretation seems to be a plausible interpretation of underdescribed procreative motives.

Procreating solely to carry on the family name, increase social status, fulfill a perceived religious or national duty, or solely for free farm labor or spare parts or marrow for existing people, while not necessarily always directly harmful to the child, does seem disrespectful of children as separate people in their own right. It is hard to imagine that procreation undertaken without any thought at all of the child as a separate and valuable person in her own right will not end up having a negative effect on the child's life (due to the negative effect on a child's well-being and self-respect that parental disrespect for the child seems likely to have). It seems reasonable to assume that, as in other areas of human behavior, motive often affects outcomes. For these reasons, procreation so motivated seems morally problematic. Note, however, that even those who procreate to maintain their family name or to provide bone marrow for a gravely ill sibling may also be motivated by a desire to love, raise, and nurture the child, that is, to engage in the parent-child relationship, once the child is born. Procreation is complex and can be multiply motivated.

Note also that those who are parentally motivated to adopt are morally similar to those who are parentally motivated to procreate biologically. One might wonder whether it is preferable, then, or even required, to adopt rather than procreate biologically since then one need not worry about the morality of creating another person at all and can even be doing good by rescuing a child from terrible prospects.[44] However, obviously, not everyone can adopt rather than procreate biologically because someone has to create the children who are adopted. Moreover, adoption is not a viable option for everyone (it's expensive and often exclusionary), and it comes at the costs of the biological joys and the biological connection, for both parent and child, that is often an aspect of biological procreativity. Further, adoption can be seen as a harsh solution to a problem that

44. See Daniel Friedrich, "A Duty to Adopt?" *Journal of Applied Philosophy* 2013 30: 25–39.

could often be more humanely resolved by enabling biological parents to care for their children. Finally, as others and I have argued elsewhere,[45] adoption is not ideal, as it often leaves children feeling abandoned and rejected and can result in parents temperamentally poorly matched with their children (this can occur with biological procreation as well, of course, though likely less frequently, given the heritability of temperament).[46] I therefore do not think that the best or only way to exercise the parental motivation is to adopt the children resulting from others' procreativity.

VI CAN WE FIND A WAY FROM HERE?

Thus we arrive at a modicum of hope. Perhaps it is possible (indeed, even ordinary) to procreate for reasons that can be characterized as something other than coercive, manipulative, and disrespectful. We have arrived at a kind of procreative motivation that we can recognize, make sense of, relate to, and not be utterly ashamed of. Still, let's not get too excited. Many problems remain. We have only taken the edge off the way

45. See Rivka Weinberg, "The Moral Complexity of Sperm Donation," *Bioethics* 2008 22: 166–178 and Velleman, "The Gift of Life." See also David Brodzinsky, *The Psychology of Adoption*, Oxford University Press, 1990; A. Jones, "Issues Relevant to Therapy with Adoptees," *Psychotherapy* 1997 34: 64–68; S. L. Nickman and A. Rosenfeld, "Children in Adoptive Families: Overview and Update," *Journal of the Academy of Child and Adolescent Psychiatry* 2005 44: 987–995; and J. J. Haugaard, A. Schustack, et al., "Birth Mothers Who Voluntarily Relinquish Infants for Adoption," *Adoption Quarterly* 1998 2: 89–97.
46. See Auke Tellegen, David Lykken, et al., "Personality Similarity in Twins Reared Apart and Together," *Journal of Personality and Social Psychology* 1988 54: 1031–1039 and the newspaper article that heralds it: *New York Times*, December 2, 1986, "Major Personality Study Finds That Traits Are Mostly Inherited."

we force people into the abyss, the way we get drunk, forget a condom, or fall in love, get married, stop using birth control, and create a human being who will have to find her way in a scary, unknown, often excruciating, brutal universe whose meaning and purpose have eluded the overwhelming majority of its inhabitants.

Wait! What happened to our modicum of hope? Let's cling to it for a moment and reflect. Perhaps we can use our understanding of procreation as an act properly motivated by the desire to engage in a unique, rich, and rewarding parent-child relationship, as a parent, yet still not undertaken for the child's sake, to further develop our procreative ethics. The parental motive may sound warm and fuzzy, and I sure hope that a good deal of parent-child relations are all about the warm fuzzies, but there is conflict inherent to procreativity. This conflict is due to the fact that whereas prospective parents have an interest in procreating—and I will elaborate on what that interest is all about in Chapter 5— no one has an interest in being born because, as argued, and as I will elaborate on in Chapter 3, all interests are contingent upon existence. Instead of an interest in existence itself, future people have an interest in an excellent or utopian existence (which is hard, if not impossible, to fulfill). I will make a case for viewing procreation as a conflict case and discuss how we best adjudicate this conflict in Chapter 5. Adjudicating the procreative conflict will require some principles of procreative ethics, formulated in Chapter 5. In Chapter 6, we will see how the procreative ethical principles arrived at in Chapter 5 apply to different kinds of procreative situations.

But we have much to attend to first. For starters, we may want to know what counts as a procreative act, who counts as having procreated, what procreative or parental responsibility entails, and how it is incurred. Getting clear on these matters will allow us to understand to whom our procreative ethical principles apply. That will be the topic of Chapter 2. And, before we apply our procreative ethical principles to anyone, we may want to investigate whether we need nuanced or complex principles at all. That's because many view life as so good as to render procreativity nearly always permissible. On this view, since most lives are worth living, the only standard of procreative care that we can support is the "life worth living" standard. That is the standard set by the non-identity problem. It is a counterintuitive, low standard. In Chapter 3, I will discuss how to avoid this low standard. I argued earlier that we can set the non-identity problem aside when discussing procreative ethics and I believe that we can, for the reasons stated earlier. However, exploring solutions to the non-identity problem can help illuminate some important issues in procreative ethics, can prove that we are not setting aside an unsolvable and compelling procreative puzzle, and can help ensure our not getting bogged down in non-identity concerns further down the road. I will offer and analyze ethical, metaphysical, and practical solutions to the non-identity problem in Chapter 3.

Just as some argue that life is so wonderful as to render almost all procreation permissible since the future child will likely have a life worth living, others argue that life is, on the whole, a bad experience. On this more melancholic view, procreating is almost always wrong because it forces a person into a bad situation (life), without the person's permission. I will address these important views in Chapter 4.

Once we are clear on what parental responsibility entails, who has it, and how one gets it (Chapter 2), and once we have analyzed whether procreation is almost always right (Chapter 3) or almost always wrong (Chapter 4), we will be ready to develop our principles of procreative ethics (Chapter 5) and discuss some applications and implications of our principles (Chapter 6).

We will have then solved the beginnings of all human difficulties—that is, being born—and can die, or end, happy.

Who Is the Parent?

(What Parental Responsibility Is and How It Is Incurred)

Before we develop our theory of procreative ethics, we will want to know whom this theory is guiding. Who bears the moral weight of creating another person? Who is the parent and which responsibilities come along with the parental role? Note that parental responsibility is not the same thing as parental rights. I make no claims here about parental rights except to note that parental rights may derive from parental responsibility and usually are assigned to those who are parentally responsible.[1]

In this chapter, I will begin with a brief analysis of what parental responsibility entails, and I will then proceed to analyze some contemporary theories about how parental responsibility is incurred. All the prevailing theories have appeal in some way, but I will argue that they are all too flawed to accept. I will then propose a Hazmat Theory of how parental responsibility is incurred, based on my view of our relationship to our hazardous gametes, and discuss some objections to and implications of the Hazmat Theory of parental responsibility.[2]

1. For an illuminating discussion of parental rights, see Harry Brighouse and Adam Swift, "Parents' Rights and the Value of the Family," *Ethics* 2006 117: 80–108.
2. I originally formulated most of the arguments in this chapter in "The Moral Complexity of Sperm Donation," *Bioethics* 2008 22: 166–178.

We will note that my theory assigns parental responsibility to gamete donors, who are currently held by many not to have incurred parental responsibility. However, I will show that they have. If we compare intentional sperm donation with accidental fatherhood (as a result of birth control failure), it is common to view the accidental father as having parental responsibility and to view the sperm donor as not having parental responsibility. The Hazmat Theory will hold both the sperm donor and the accidental father parentally responsible for their offspring. In fact, I will show that none of the currently prevailing theories of how parental responsibility is incurred can make sense of the view that the sperm donor is not parentally responsible but the accidental father is. So the fact that the Hazmat Theory of parental responsibility cannot accommodate that set of intuitions either is no reason to reject the theory—you will not do any better by the contradictory set of intuitions about parental responsibility on prevailing alternate theories. No theory will accommodate the contradictory set of intuitions, so we will have to give up one of them. I will argue that rather than deem accidental fathers free of parental responsibility, we should consider gamete donors parentally responsible, as implied by the Hazmat Theory of parental responsibility. We can then consider whether parental responsibility can be transferred and, if so, under what sorts of conditions.

I PARENTAL RESPONSIBILITY

Parental responsibility is the responsibility to play the parental role in a child's life.[3] To properly play a parental role, one must

---

3. Like most responsibilities, if you have a responsibility that you're not able to fulfill yourself, you are responsible to see to it that the responsibility is fulfilled, to the extent possible, by someone else.

raise and nurture one's child. Nurturing a child generally involves attending to her needs, helping her grow into her own person, and guiding her toward an appropriate and productive adulthood in the course of a caring and loving relationship. Why the love? Because that's what is needed in order for a child to grow into a healthy, productive adult—a long-term loving relationship with a nurturing caregiver. While there are surely some exceptionally resilient children who grow into healthy productive adults even in the absence of a long-term nurturing relationship with a caregiver, the attachment and developmental difficulties that children who lack sustained nurturing caregivers experience argue in favor of requiring parents to love, raise, and nurture their children toward adulthood.[4] Being the caregiver in a caring and loving long-term relationship with a child is what parental responsibility entails, although a good deal (though not nearly all) of the caregiving is appropriately delegated to others, like doctors, teachers, babysitters, and so on. That's what parental responsibility is. So how do you get (or avoid) it?

II HOW PARENTAL RESPONSIBILITY IS INCURRED: PREVAILING THEORIES

(i) Voluntary Commitments Some people explicitly volunteer for parental responsibility and are then widely considered to be

---

4. See Zeanah, McLaughlin et al., "Attachment as a Mechanism Linking Foster Care Placement to Improved Mental Health Outcomes in Previously Institutionalized Children," *Journal of Child Psychology and Psychiatry* 2012 53: 46–55; Judith Solomon and Carol George, "The Disorganized Attachment Caregiving System: Dysregulation of Adaptive Processes at Multiple Levels," in *Disorganized Attachment and Caregiving*, Solomon and George, Eds., Guilford Press, 2011, 3–24; and David Howe, "Attachment: Assessing Children's Needs and Parenting Capacity," in *The Child's World: The Comprehensive Guide to Assessing Children in Need*, 2nd ed., Jessica Kingsley Publishers, 2010, 184–198; among many others.

parentally responsible for their children. Adoption is an example of voluntary commitments resulting in parental responsibility. Like any promise or commitment, the promise or commitment to be parentally responsible for a child will usually obligate a person to fulfill this commitment. But simply stating that it is our voluntary commitments that make us parentally responsible is uninformative because it says little about what counts as a voluntary commitment of this kind. In fact, one way of framing the question of parental responsibility would be to ask what counts as a voluntary parental commitment. Do I have to sign on the dotted line or just have sex without a condom? If this theory requires an explicit commitment to parenthood, then we will be left with many children without anyone responsible to raise them since it does not take an explicit commitment to raise a child in order to create a child. On the other hand, if it takes little to be considered to have voluntarily committed to parental responsibility, then we may find ourselves with many competing claims to parenthood. Because the voluntary commitment theory of parental responsibility does not tell us what counts as a voluntary commitment, it is uninformative at best. At worst, it leaves many children with no one parentally responsible for them and/or many competing parties with the ability to claim parental responsibility (and the rights that come along with it). Hopefully, we can do better than too many parents, too few parents, or a huge question mark in lieu of parents.

(ii) Intent to Raise Some argue that parental responsibility belongs to the people who have the parental intent, that is, to the people who intend to play the caretaking parental role.[5] This

---

5. See J. L. Hill, "'What Does It Mean to Be a Parent?': The Claims of Biology as the Basis for Parental Rights," *New York University Law Review* 1991 66: 353–420.

claim is usually presented in the context of a surrogacy dispute, in order to support the claims of the nonbiological parent against the genetic or gestative claims of the surrogate.[6] Like the voluntary commitments theory, the intent-to-raise theory can leave many children with no one parentally responsible for them,[7] and it has some additional problems: intentions can change,[8] and anyone can claim to be parentally responsible by claiming intent. The intent can be both outlandish and genuine at the same time—I can genuinely intend to raise the second child of the second couple to inhabit the second story of the apartment building across the street from my second home, but that is no reason to think that my inexplicable intention makes me parentally responsible for that child. Even worse, anyone can deny responsibility by denying intent: I can seek out unprotected intercourse intentionally timed for an optimal chance at conception, get pregnant, birth the child, and genuinely deny that I ever intended to raise the child. If we base responsibility on intent, we allow people to decide what is attributable to them since we often cannot know another's intention.[9] Here too, I hope we can do better than too many parents, too few parents, or a huge question mark in lieu of parents.

(iii) Gestationalism It has been claimed that the person who gestates the child is the person parentally responsible for the

---

6. See the literature on the Mary Beth Whitehead case. *In the Matter of Baby M* 109 N.J. 396, 537 A. 2nd (N.J. 1988).

7. As many have noted. See Elizabeth Anderson, "Is Women's Labor a Commodity?" *Philosophy and Public Affairs* 1990 19: 71–92; and Tim Bayne and Avery Kolers, "Toward a Pluralistic Account of Parenthood," *Bioethics* 2003 17: 221–242; among others.

8. See Melinda Roberts, "Good Intentions and a Great Divide: Having Babies by Intending Them," *Law and Philosophy* 1983 12: 287–317.

9. See Arthur Ripstein, *Equality, Responsibility, and the Law*, Cambridge University Press, 1996.

child. This claim is usually made by those intending to protect the rights of surrogate mothers (since it is usually the person with parental responsibility who is also accorded corresponding parental rights). On this view, fatherhood is derived from a man's relationship to the woman who gestates the fetus and not directly from his relationship to the child. Thus, without any compelling rationale, fatherhood is reduced to derivative status only.[10] Proponents of gestationalism argue that the risk, labor, and discomfort of gestation, as well as the love and attachment that develop between gestator and baby during gestation, ground claims to parental rights and the concomitant responsibilities.[11] But this view is riddled with problems: First, it seems more aimed at parental rights than at parental responsibilities. Second, claiming parental rights to a child on the basis of one's risk and labor investment implies commodification since risk and labor investment are the ways we justify claims to property. Third, although feelings of attachment may develop during pregnancy, they may not develop in the gestator, and they may develop in others who may feel a growing attachment to the baby even though they are not gestating it.

Without a compelling argument, and none has been provided, there seems no reason to accept that gestating alone is the determinant of parental responsibility, especially because it is at least theoretically possible that, one day, no person will gestate babies. Instead, babies may be gestated by sophisticated

---

10. See Bayne and Kolers, "Toward a Pluralistic Account."
11. See Uma Narayan, "Family Ties: Rethinking Parental Claims in the Light of Surrogacy and Custody," in *Having and Raising Children: Unconventional Families, Hard Choices, and the Social Good*, Narayan and Julia J. Bartkowiak, Eds., Pennsylvania State University Press, 1999; Barbara Rothman, *Recreating Motherhood: Ideology and Technology in a Patriarchal Society*, Norton, 1989; and Susan Feldman, "Multiple Biological Mothers: The Case for Gestation," *Journal of Social Philosophy* 1992 23: 98–104.

incubators. There are already babies born today who have spent nearly as much time developing in incubators as they did in uteruses (babies born at twenty-two to twenty-four weeks gestation sometimes survive). Would no one be parentally responsible for such babies? Gestationalism denies fathers direct parental responsibility, could possibly grant parental responsibility to no one, provides us with no good reason to accept it as a theory of parental responsibility, and seems like little more than an ad hoc attempt to bolster surrogates' claims in contested surrogacy cases. Therefore, we should reject it as a theory of parental responsibility.

(iv) Causation One intuitive way to determine responsibility is to try to figure out who caused the child to exist in the first place. On this view, by causing the existence of a helpless baby or by being responsible for the creation of the child's needs, one becomes (parentally) responsible to equip, guide, and nurture the child through the minefield of life. When we see a needy baby, it makes sense for us to ask, "Who caused this needy baby?" and the answer to that question seems to finger the person responsible to take care of the needy baby. But it fingers too many people.[12] It can point to fertility specialists, eager grandparents, the friends who brought that fabulous bottle of wine to dinner, and so on. Is that too far a stretch? You might think that, like obscenity, causation is hard to define but we know it when we see it. Lindemann-Nelson argues along these lines:

> A pair of coordinated actions which were proximate to and jointly sufficient for some event, and were not the result of

12. See Ripstein, *Equality*, 35–36.

forcing or fraudulent action on the part of others would be hard not to see as *the* cause of the event in question. Becoming a parent generally fits this model.[13]

However, many parents' coordinated actions are not jointly sufficient for the birth of their child since they require medical assistance to conceive, gestate, or birth a child. In fact, biological parents are probably never causally sufficient for the creation of their child since so many factors determine conception, gestation, and birth. Even though biological parents are usually "irreplaceably involved"[14] in their child's creation in ways that other people aren't, this by itself does not make them the "real" cause, the proximate cause, or even the sufficient cause. Grandparents, doctors, boring TV writers, whoever caused the blackout, whoever brought the wine to dinner, may be causally necessary for the child's existence. Some of these people may have also been irreplaceably involved in the child's creation. A very insistent and influential grandparent can be more causally or irreplaceably involved in the creation of a child than the child's more passive, eager-to-please parents. Is the grandparent then the one with parental responsibility for the child? Despite its intuitive appeal, causation spreads parental responsibility too widely,[15] and it can also miss its intended targets. It would be better if we could find a theory free of these defects.

---

13. James Lindemann-Nelson, "Parental Obligations and the Ethics of Surrogacy: A Causal Perspective," *Public Affairs Quarterly* 1991 5: 49–61.
14. Nelson, "Parental Obligations."
15. Giuliana Fuscaldo argues that parental responsibility is held by *all* who voluntarily and foreseeably contribute to a child's existence. This widespread sort of responsibility, which is claimed to vary in degree and in kind, is not what I mean by *parental* responsibility. See Giuliana Fuscaldo, "Genetic Ties: Are They Morally Binding?" *Bioethics* 2006 20: 64–76.

(v) Geneticism People are biological organisms, created biologically. Biologically speaking, the person whose genetic material is transferred or copied to create another being is the new being's parent. This holds true for all kinds of organisms, from the most simple to the most complex. When a single-celled organism splits into two cells, the resulting two single-celled organisms are called the "daughter" cells of the original cell. Similarly, we can call the organism formed from the gamete cells of two people the child of those people, no? To a large extent, it has been argued, we do so already in our social and legal practices, which implicitly endorse geneticism by requiring sperm donors, egg donors, and surrogate mothers to transfer or waive their parental rights and responsibilities.[16] If geneticism were not assumed, gamete donors and surrogate mothers would have no rights or responsibilities to transfer or waive. But this only shows that geneticism is frequently assumed. It doesn't show that the assumption is warranted. And there have been numerous challenges to geneticism, mostly centered on the problem of voluntariness. If someone forcibly steals your gametes, it is hard to see how you can be deemed responsible for any resulting offspring.[17] Because it is generally unfair to hold people responsible for things beyond what is reasonably thought to be in their control, when seeking to determine parental responsibility, geneticism cannot be the whole story.

16. See Edgar Page, "Donation, Surrogacy, and Adoption," *Journal of Applied Philosophy* 1985 2: 161–172.
17. See Tim Bayne, "Gamete Donation and Parental Responsibility," *Journal of Applied Philosophy* 2003 20: 77–87; David Benatar, "The Unbearable Lightness of Bringing into Being," *Journal of Applied Philosophy* 1999 16: 173–180; Jeffrey Blustein, "Procreation and Parental Responsibility," *Journal of Social Philosophy* 1997 28: 80–82; and Jeff McMahan, *The Ethics of Killing: Problems at the Margins of Life*, Oxford University Press, 2002, 374.

(vi) Hybrids To complete what geneticism leaves out, Benatar's view of parental responsibility can be seen as a combination of geneticism and some element of voluntarism. He argues that reproductive autonomy entails the right to make reproductive decisions about whether to procreate and also confers responsibility for the results of having this right. He deems this to be the case even when it is not clear that this right is being exercised, for example, in cases of thoughtless or accidental procreation, because he holds people responsible for their failure to responsibly engage their reproductive autonomy.[18] When control is transferred, for example, in cases of sperm or gonad donation, parental responsibility is transferred as well.

According to Benatar, reproductive autonomy entails parental responsibility for unforced use of one's reproductive capacities. But he does not define reproductive autonomy, and it's therefore unclear how to assess the view. Are people who use fairly reliable birth control but conceive anyway parentally responsible? They have exercised their reproductive autonomy but they were exercising it in ways aimed at preventing parental responsibility. Does that matter? Benatar holds people responsible for thoughtless pregnancy due to their failure to engage their reproductive autonomy in a responsible way. Does this mean that people who do engage their reproductive autonomy responsibly, for example, by using the pill, are released from presumptive parental responsibility? Without knowing how or why reproductive autonomy entails parental responsibility, it is hard to know which choices or acts are the ones that generate parental responsibility, and it also seems like we may well be left with children who have no one parentally responsible for them.

18. Benatar, "Unbearable Lightness."

Bayne and Kolers argue for a pluralistic account of parental responsibility that incorporates the various causal elements that contribute to the creation of a child.[19] On their view, although neither intent nor gestation nor genetic ties are necessary for parental responsibility, each may be sufficient to generate parental responsibility because each of those elements can often be causally linked to child creation. That is why they think that an account of parental responsibility "ought to be broad enough to grant parenthood to genetic, gestational, custodial, and intentional parents."[20]

The upside of pluralism is that little is left out. The downside, here, is the opposite. With little left out, too much is included. When so many people are eligible for parental responsibility, we have no way to decide who is and who is not parentally responsible, and to what degree. Parental responsibility is spread too broadly by granting it to genetic, gestational, custodial, and intentional parents because when different people play these roles and can claim or disclaim responsibility, how are we to decide which claims are legitimate? It seems consistent with this view to hold all parties responsible, but do we really want to say that one child can have sixteen parents, all with equal levels of parental responsibility (and the rights often deemed to come along with it)? That may seem to give children more protection, but it can also turn out to give them less: with so many candidates for parental responsibility, children may be left with no one particularly parentally responsible for them since no criterion for parental responsibility is given priority over another. By fingering so many possibly responsible people and giving us no clear way of distinguishing levels of

19. Bayne and Kolers, "Toward a Pluralistic Account."
20. Bayne and Kolers, "Toward a Pluralistic Account."

responsibility among them, each candidate can point to another, leaving the child with no one. We also need to justify saddling so many people with so weighty a responsibility. Simply being somehow causally related to the fact that there's a new child in town is not enough of a justification.

Hybrid theories attempt to respond to the complexity of parental responsibility with more nuance and fluidity. This may sound like a good strategy, but it does not work out so well pragmatically. We want to avoid diffusing parental responsibility to the point where it seems to slip away altogether.

III   HOW PARENTAL RESPONSIBILITY IS REALLY INCURRED: THE HAZMAT THEORY OF PARENTAL RESPONSIBILITY

Here is how parental responsibility happens: You own and control some dangerous stuff. You have to take care of it because it could really hurt someone. If you don't make sure it doesn't blow up or if you intentionally set off an explosion, you have to pay for the cleanup and/or enjoy the fireworks (depending on how happy you are to be parentally responsible). This is consistent with our moral and legal views regarding our responsibility for the risks we take and impose with the hazardous materials under our possession and control, and for the behavior we choose to engage in with them. If you own a car, which is a dangerous possession, and you choose to drive it (carefully) in the rain, if you skid into a pedestrian who is crossing the street in accordance with traffic laws and she breaks her leg, you are responsible to mitigate the damage incurred by the risks you chose to take with the dangerous possession under your possession and control. Similarly, if you own some gametes, and you engage in behavior that allows them to join with others and grow into a child who will suffer great harm unless she is properly cared for, you are responsible to mitigate the damage incurred by the risks you chose to take with the dangerous possessions under your possession and control.

Parental responsibility derives from our possession and high degree of control over our gametes, which are a form of hazardous material. Our gametes are hazardous because they can join with the gametes of others and grow into extremely needy innocent persons with full moral status. Being in possession and control of such hazardous material is a very serious responsibility. Gametes are a high-risk material and that risk demands a high standard of care. It's like owning a pet lion or inheriting lots of enriched uranium. You can't just leave that sort of stuff lying around. Dangerous possessions under our voluntary control, for example, enriched uranium, a loaded gun, young ripe ova, or viable sperm, generate a very high standard of care. If we do things that put our gametes at risk of joining with others and growing into persons, we assume the costs (and rewards) of that risky activity.

Let us take a moment to think about risk and responsibility. Risky activities are usually engaged in because someone wants to engage in them. The risky activities often put other people in harm's way. For example, you may want to enjoy the thrill of driving quickly in a downpour, but that puts the people in the other cars on the road at risk of your crashing into them. We can view this as a conflict of interests between the risk imposer and the risk imposee. The imposer has an interest in freely engaging in activities of her choice and the imposee has an interest in avoiding becoming a victim of a risk that results in harm. It seems fair to adjudicate this conflict of interests by weighing the cost to each party of having the other party's interests prevail. (In this case, we would weigh the cost of being restricted in your speed while driving in a downpour versus the cost of being hit by another car while you are both driving in the rain.) It is a reasonable way to establish the relative strength of the competing claims that, in turn, helps to establish the standard of care for that kind of activity.[21]

Not all risky activities generate a high standard of care. When we breathe we risk communicating diseases, but we don't usually hold exhalers responsible for the harm that may result from their risky breathing activity. We usually judge the exhalers' interests in breathing freely to be stronger than the inhalers' interests in avoiding a cold because the costs of not exhaling are usually steeper than the costs of occasionally becoming infected from someone else's exhalation. However, if someone knows that she has a very serious and highly contagious flu, she has no business visiting someone with a compromised immune system and exhaling flu all over that person. Owning a pet lion is another clear case in which the interests of your neighbors in avoiding being lion lunch trump your interests in owning a pet lion.

What about gamete-releasing activities? It seems to me that the costs (to the child) of being born without specific people highly responsible and committed to one's care are far more serious than the costs (to the parents) of being restricted from cost-free engagement in behavior that risks creating a child from one's gametes. This doesn't mean that engaging in behavior that risks the creation of a child from one's gametes is therefore wrong or reckless. It just means that the costs of engaging in risky behavior with one's gametes belong to those who engage in it.[22] Parental

---

21. See Ripstein, *Equality*, Chapters 1 and 3.
22. Here, for the most part, I follow Ripstein's liability analysis model, *Equality*, 70–72.

responsibility is a cost (or reward) of the risks we choose to take with the hazardous gametes we possess. Parental responsibility is incurred when we choose to engage in activities that put our gametes at risk of joining with others and growing into persons, and persons result from those activities. That is the Hazmat Theory of parental responsibility.

Note that the Hazmat Theory tells us how parental responsibility is incurred but does not set the procreative standard of care more generally—meaning, it does not tell us which procreative risks we may impose on our children—and it does not tell us when we can permissibly procreate. No one can be absolutely sure that she will be able to fulfill her parental responsibilities since anyone can die anytime, or become incapacitated, homeless, and so on. So we will not set absolute standards of procreative care because that would impose too high a cost on parents. No one would be able to procreate if the ability to fulfill one's parental responsibilities had to be absolutely guaranteed. But we won't set very low standards either, for example, allowing impoverished, mentally ill adolescents to procreate, because that would impose too high a cost on the children. But I am getting way too far ahead of myself. We will figure out how to set a reasonable standard of procreative care over the course of this book, mostly in Chapter 5, by thinking about the costs to parents of being restricted from procreativity and the costs to children posed by a lack of such procreative constraints. What we are focused on in this chapter is figuring out when and how parental responsibility is incurred at all. The Hazmat Theory tells us that the initial standard of care for our gametes is very high—we can't just play around with them willy-nilly because if they join with others and become persons, then we are parentally responsible for those persons.

(i) Advantages of the Hazmat Theory The Hazmat Theory provides us with a rationale for parental responsibility that is consistent with the ways in which we hold people responsible for risky activity and dangerous possessions under their control. It fits the procreative act into our system of moral, legal, and societal norms governing the standard of care we assign to those in possession and control of dangerous things and risky activity. This is something that the competing theories don't even attempt, lending them all an air of ad hoc-ness.

The Hazmat Theory of parental responsibility is consistent with many of our intuitions regarding the high level of responsibility we tend to think we have for the children who result from our gametes. It explains why we hold people parentally responsible for children who result from birth control failure, drunken or half-conscious activity, and unbridled passion. It explains why people are parentally responsible for their so-called unintended children, but it also explains why we think that one is not parentally responsible for the children that result from one's stolen testicle.[23] It explains why we don't think that fertility doctors are usually parentally responsible: unlike gamete owners, fertility doctors don't possess rights of ownership and control over the gametes they are paid to manipulate.[24] It even explains why we hold people responsible for their staggering stupidity ("I didn't know you could get pregnant while . . ." Fill in the blank: breastfeeding, standing up, postpartum, perimenopausal, fifteen, etc.). When it comes to hazardous materials, ignorance of how to use

---

23. A donated testicle, however, would likely be considered by the Hazmat Theory to be a case of mass sperm donation.
24. Fertility doctors and professionals may have special professional and moral responsibilities, but they do not have *parental* responsibilities, even though they are often crucial actors in the process of the creation of a child.

them safely is often no excuse for unwanted outcomes because part of the responsibility we have for the hazardous materials we own and control is the responsibility to learn how to properly safeguard them.

The Hazmat Theory avoids the pitfalls of the competing prevailing theories of parental responsibility. It doesn't leave many children with no one parentally responsible for them (as the voluntary commitments and intent theories do and as gestationalism and Bayne and Kolers' pluralistic theory could); it doesn't leave children with so many people possibly parentally responsible for them as to be practically not viable when we are trying to determine parental responsibility (as the causation and Bayne and Kolers' pluralistic theories do); it doesn't hold people responsible for actions well beyond their control (as geneticism can); and it is not indeterminate regarding which actions generate parental responsibility (as Benatar's reproductive autonomy theory can be).

It's not a perfect theory, but it's pretty good at explaining when, how, and why parental responsibility is incurred (and it does a better job than the alternative theories). I will now address some objections to the Hazmat Theory of parental responsibility.

(ii)   Objections to the Hazmat Theory

a) *I Never Asked for Gametes!* Of course, there's a difference between owning a pet lion and finding oneself a possessor of a steady supply of gametes. We can choose not to own a lion. That's the choice most of us would take, given the high level of responsibility we would incur by owning a lion. But we are born with gametes lurking within us, primed to bolt and join with others.

It's what they do. Yet it is not the bare fact of our (involuntary) ownership of our gametes that makes us parentally responsible for the results of their union with others. It is the risks we choose to take with them. The risks we choose to take with our gametes are what makes us parentally responsible for what happens to them, should they develop into needy beings with full moral status. However, because we are born with gametes and have a high interest in procreating, the standard of procreative care will not be a strict liability standard (the standard we apply to pet lion ownership). Meaning, while we are parentally responsible to the children who grow from the gametes under our jurisdiction, we are not responsible to compensate our children for every burden that befalls them. Parental responsibility entails the obligation to raise, love, and nurture one's child to adulthood, but it does not entail the obligation to compensate her for anything bad that happens to her. (More on this in Chapter 5, section VI.) If we want to avoid parental responsibility, we can abstain from sexual intercourse, use two highly reliable methods of birth control simultaneously, or surgically interfere with our gamete-release system.

b) *Causing Need Doesn't Necessarily Obligate One to Meet the Need:* In the context of the abortion debate, it has been argued that causing a need does not automatically or necessarily obligate you to meet that need.[25] So why assume that causing a child's needs obligates you to meet her needs? This objection is misplaced here—the Hazmat Theory makes no such assumptions about causation and responsibility for needs. It is not a causal theory of parental responsibility, and it does not ground parental

25. See McMahan, *The Ethics of Killing,* 364–372.

responsibility in claims regarding obligations to meet needs one caused or created per se. The Hazmat Theory is based on the responsibilities we have regarding the risks we take and impose with the dangerous things under our possession and control. It is grounded in our moral and legal theories of responsibility for hazardous property, negligence, and risk imposition (as discussed above).

c) *Gamete Theft:* What about rape or gamete theft? If someone rapes you or steals your gametes, it is the rapist or the gamete thief who bears the cost of the risky gamete behavior since it is they, and not you, who voluntarily engaged in activities that risk having gametes under their control unite to form a person. You may still have obligations and responsibilities to the child, but they will not be parental ones.[26]

d) *Hazmat Ignores Gestational, Intentional, and Voluntary Commitments:* The Hazmat Theory does not give special weight to genetic, gestational, or intentional ties, and these bonds are important. Yet the Hazmat Theory does not deny their importance. It just denies that these sorts of connections give rise to parental responsibilities. It does not deny that they may be important in many respects and may give rise to various sorts of responsibilities.

e) *Hazmat Makes Fathers Out of Sperm Donors and Mothers Out of Egg Donors!* Many people think that gamete donors are not parentally responsible for the children who result from their gametes. The Hazmat Theory seems to hold gamete donors parentally

---

26. For example, if you birth a child born of rape, you may not be parentally responsible for the child, but you are at least as responsible as you might be to any newborn in your sphere of control (e.g., to bring the child to the orphanage or to the attention of social services, etc.).

responsible for their offspring. How can that be right? A set of examples will help illustrate how that can be right:

Meet the Joes

Joe Blow:

Joe Blow has a one-night stand with Jane, using the just-in-case condom he carries in his wallet. It is a brand-name, unexpired condom that, unbeknownst to Joe, has a very tiny hole in it. Jane gets pregnant and gives birth to Jack. Joe walks away. He refuses to give any time, attention, or money to Jack.

Joe Spermdonor:

Joe Spermdonor completes an application to donate sperm to an agency. He is deemed a desirable donor. He donates sperm, accepts the standard monetary compensation, and goes home. His sperm is inserted into Sheila who gets pregnant and gives birth to Julie. Joe Spermdonor never meets Julie and does not support or parent her at all.

When confronted with this set of cases, it is common to want to find some way to hold Joe Blow parentally responsible for Jack but release Joe Spermdonor from responsibility for Julie.[27] This desire, like so many others, will have to go unfulfilled. No

---

27. In the United States, a sperm donor is not usually considered to be the "natural father" of the resulting child. In most states in the United States, where the natural father usually has initial parental responsibility, if the sperm recipient is a married woman, her husband is considered the legal, initial father of the child (not the adoptive father). "The donor of semen provided to a licensed physician for use in artificial insemination of a woman other than the donor's wife is treated in law as if he were not the natural father of a child thereby conceived" (Cal. Civil Code § 7005[b]). Note that if the sperm donation is not done via an official process or with a licensed doctor or agency, the sperm donor may be held parentally responsible by law. See, "Kansas Man Who Donated Sperm to Lesbian Couple Being Sued by State for Child Support," Associated Press, January 13, 2013.

theory of parental responsibility can support this contradictory set of intuitions. We will have to give one up. Giving up the intuition that Joe Spermdonor is not parentally responsible for Julie is less counterintuitive and more supported by our theoretical commitments than is giving up the intuition that Joe Blow is not parentally responsible for Jack. (If Joe Blow is not parentally responsible for Jack, we have to reject centuries of cross-cultural legal and social views regarding paternity and paternal parental responsibility.) So letting sperm donors off the hook is the belief that's got to go.

First, let us distinguish between responsibility to the adults with whom one procreates and responsibility to the child one creates. These responsibilities are often conflated, but they are, in fact, separate. When two people voluntarily engage in activity that risks creating a child, it seems reasonable to expect both of them to bear responsibility for the results. In cases of sperm or egg donation (or, more typically, sale), the recipient (or buyer) of the sperm or ova agrees to absolve the donor (or seller) of parental responsibility. This may release the sperm donor (or seller) of the responsibility he would otherwise have to the mother of his child and release the egg donor (or seller) of the responsibility she would otherwise have to the father of her child, but it does not release anyone from parental responsibility to the child. Obligations to the adults with whom one procreates are separate from obligations to the children one procreates. Fulfilling your obligations to one doesn't thereby fulfill them to the other.

Now let's look at how each theory of parental responsibility would treat the Joes:

Voluntary commitments will not distinguish between the Joes. It will hold neither Joe Blow nor Joe Spermdonor parentally responsible since neither of them voluntarily committed to be parentally responsible. Intent to raise will not distinguish between the Joes either. It will hold neither Joe parentally responsible since neither of them intended to raise his child. Gestationalism will also draw no distinction between the Joes and hold neither of them parentally responsible since neither of them gestated his child and neither of them is in a relationship with the woman who gestated his child.

Causation will not help us distinguish between the Joes either. It will hold them both parentally responsible since they are both crucial causes of their child's existence. Though neither is a sufficient cause of his child's existence, both are necessary causes of their (respective) child's existence. Joe Spermdonor, however, is a slightly less proximate cause of his child's existence than Joe Blow is of his since Joe Spermdonor does not actually impregnate anyone. But that slight difference in physical proximity does not diminish Joe Spermdonor's crucial causal role in his child's existence.[28] The fact that Joe Spermdonor does not insert the sperm into Sheila himself does not make him any less necessarily or voluntarily a cause, only slightly less proximate, much as fathers whose wives are artificially inseminated with their sperm are slightly less proximate a cause of their resulting child. You don't need to be the direct proximate cause of something in order to be a causal agent, and the mere presence of an intervening link in an intentional, foreseeable causal chain does not diminish causal agency. If I kill you myself, I am the proximate causal agent of your death; if I hire a hitman to kill you, I'm no longer the most proximate causal agent

28. See Ronald Munson, "Artificial Insemination and Donor Responsibility," in *Intention and Reflection: Basic Issues in Bioethics*, Wadsworth, 1988.

of your death (just as Joe Spermdonor hasn't impregnated anyone, I haven't killed anyone), but I am still a causal agent of your death and probably the most important one. So even if the causal account of parental responsibility were correct, it would not draw a moral distinction between our two Joes.

Geneticism, of course, can't distinguish between the Joes. It holds them both parentally responsible for their genetic offspring.

Whether Benatar's hybrid theory distinguishes between the two Joes depends upon which decisions are considered to be reproductively autonomous. On the most obvious interpretation, both Joes are parentally responsible because both make voluntary reproductive decisions yielding a child who results from their gametes: Joe Blow decides to have sex with a less than foolproof contraceptive; Joe Spermdonor decides to donate sperm to be used to create a child. I think that is the correct application of Benatar's view to this set of cases. However, one could argue that if we are taking reproductive autonomy seriously, Joe Blow has a lesser degree of responsibility because had his reproductively autonomous choice had its usual and intended effect, he would not have created a child. But that interpretation takes us further from the common intuitions we were trying to support.

Bayne and Kolers' pluralistic account of parental responsibility won't help us either. If it tells us anything about our Joes at all, it seems most likely to hold them both parentally responsible since they both satisfy the genetic criteria, deemed sufficient for parental responsibility by this theory, and neither satisfies the gestational, intentional, or custodial criteria. If either is held more parentally responsible than the other, it is likely to be Joe Spermdonor since he comes closer to being an intentional parent (by donating sperm to be used to create a child) than does Joe Blow, giving him two criteria to Joe Blow's one.

No theory of parental responsibility can support the intuition that Joe Blow is parentally responsible for Jack but Joe Spermdonor is not parentally responsible for Julie. The Hazmat Theory can't do it either, but it can explain why Joe Blow is responsible for Jack, even though Joe Blow is not especially reckless and did not intend to father a child. The Hazmat Theory holds both Joes parentally responsible for the risks they took with their hazardous materials. Joe Blow should know that sperm often breach the condom gate (it says so on the condom wrapper). Joe Spermdonor donates his sperm to a brokering agency for the express purpose of procreation (it says so in the contract). Since both Joes voluntarily engage in activities that put their respective gametes at risk of joining with others and growing into persons and persons result from their respective activities, both Joes are parentally responsible for those resulting persons.

IV CAN PARENTAL RESPONSIBILITY BE TRANSFERRED?

If parental responsibility can be responsibly transferred, then having it in the first place is less burdensome. There are two kinds of transfer to consider: transfer of the initial responsibility and transfer of the current, ongoing responsibility.

(i) Transferring Initial Parental Responsibility We may wonder whether transfer of gamete ownership and control transfers (initial) parental responsibility since it transfers the source or reason for the responsibility. We might think that this is what happens when someone donates gametes. Maybe that's what

happens when Joe Spermdonor transfers his hazardous materials to the sperm bank or to Sheila, via the sperm bank.[29] That would be surprising, though, because the very high standard of care that we have for our gametes will not easily accommodate a transfer of responsibility. Imagine if I decide to sell my cache of enriched uranium to a uranium brokering agency. Surely that won't absolve me of responsibility for the nuclear explosion that may result (especially if I know that the mission of the brokering agency is to sell the enriched uranium to people who want to use it to create controlled explosions). Enriched uranium is so volatile and dangerous that it is not easy to safely and reliably transfer it. In order to really transfer responsibility for my enriched uranium to someone else, I'd have to transfer it very carefully, to a very reputable agent, and for a very good reason. Extreme care, caution, and investigation would be required. Current practices of sperm and ova donation in many countries, including the United States, fall far short of any claim to the very high standard of care that transferring such hazardous material would demand.[30] Anonymous gamete donation, clearly, does not meet a high standard of care in transferring hazardous materials since you don't even know whom you're transferring it to and the agencies you sell to exist not to investigate potential customers but to make a profit by selling gametes. Anonymous gamete donation (or sale) is a reckless use

---

29. I am grateful to Masahiro Yamada for raising this question.
30. Although the precise standard of care is not set out here, since sperm donors in many countries currently have no information about where their sperm is going, there cannot be any claim to investigation or significant care at all. Therefore, the current practice usually does not even meet a moderate standard of care, let alone any standard of care that can claim to be high. A similar point is made by Benatar. See Benatar, "Unbearable Lightness," 176.

of one's hazardous materials.[31] It falls woefully short of the high standard of care that ownership and control over hazardous material demand.

The difficulty with claiming that transferring ownership and control over one's gametes makes the recipients the ones with initial parental responsibility for the children who result from them runs much deeper than current gamete-donation procedures. Arguably, donating sperm or ova is not simply a *transfer* of ownership and control but, rather, is an *exercise* of the donor's ownership and control, for purposes of uniting his gamete with another's (usually, for a cash bonus). Sperm donors take the gametes that they own and control and give them to someone else for procreative purposes, much like ordinary fathers do (except for the cash bonus). Egg donors take the gametes that they own and control and give them to someone else for procreative purposes, differing from ordinary mothers only in not gestating their fetuses, which is not necessary for parental responsibility anyway, as argued earlier.

It might be argued that, unlike sperm or egg donors, ordinary mothers and fathers don't waive parental rights and are not supposedly absolved of parental responsibility. But waiving one's parental rights and being supposedly absolved of parental responsibility by the gamete recipient seems, if anything, to confirm one's initial parental responsibility. If you are not initially responsible, you have no responsibility to transfer and no rights to waive. Gamete donors may claim to have transferred their responsibility

---

31. Even though those who buy gametes want children and can afford to buy gametes, we know that the desire for children and the means to buy gametes are no indication of mental stability, kindness, consistency, patience, and other qualities that contribute to adequate parenting. The prevalence and persistence of child abuse and neglect make relying on intentional parenthood as some guarantee of adequate parenting completely unwarranted and, yes, reckless.

for the resulting child, but they can't claim never to have incurred that responsibility.

a) *Parent Proliferation:* In cases of irresponsible transfer of parental responsibilities, we may end up with more than two people who are parentally responsible for one child. This can occur because, as argued earlier, like any promise, the promise to be parentally responsible for a child obligates the promisor to fulfill her promise. This entails that if a sperm donor irresponsibly transfers parental responsibility to a recipient couple and that couple commits to being parentally responsible to the child resulting from that sperm, both the couple and the sperm donor are parentally responsible to the child (the sperm donor due to the Hazmat Theory of parental responsibility and the couple due to the general obligation we have to keep our promises and fulfill our commitments).[32] If a couple goes gamete shopping, as is currently legal in the United States, and buys sperm and egg from various brokers, we will have four people parentally responsible to the same child (the gamete sellers due to their initial parental responsibility and irresponsible transfer of it; the gamete buyers due to their promise and commitment to be parentally responsible to the child). This proliferation of parents may result in confusion and conflict regarding who has which responsibilities or rights associated with parental responsibilities and rights. This unfortunate result would be avoided if we adhered to the standards set by the Hazmat Theory of parental responsibility.

(ii) Transfer of Current or Ongoing Parental Responsibility What about transferring parental responsibility? Is it the kind of responsibility that can be transferred?

---

32. This scenario was suggested to me by David Wasserman.

Parental responsibility includes the responsibility to provide for one's child's basic needs. My misgivings about transferring parental responsibility are based on the premise that love is one of a child's basic needs. If a child's basic needs include the need to be loved, it is unclear to me that a responsibility of this kind—a responsibility to relate with a particular feeling toward another person—can be coherently transferred.

When we promise to love our spouses in sickness and in health, can we fulfill this promise by transferring it to someone else? "Now that you are confined to a wheelchair, I don't love you anymore, but my friend Sally is willing to" is a ridiculous attempt to fulfill one's spousal promise. And it is ridiculous because you have promised *your* love, not someone else's. It's true that disrupting a loving relationship via transfer, as I describe in this case, is worse than transferring the obligation to love before the relationship develops over time because it has the added negative element of disruption. But note that you need not already be engaged in a loving relationship in order to promise to love someone or to be obligated to love someone. Promising to love someone prior to developing a loving relationship occurs in many arranged marriages, and being obligated to love someone prior to developing a loving relationship with that person occurs in many arranged marriages and, arguably, in standard procreative cases. The duty to love generated by marital or procreative commitments is problematic to transfer not because it's disruptive to a loving relationship (although, when present, that element makes the transfer even more problematic) but, rather, because it is hard to see how we can transfer personal commitments to personally relate to another person in a particular emotional way and also because commitments to uniquely performed tasks generate an obligation to perform the task oneself (e.g., when a comedian commits to a gig, she can't just send another comedian in her stead).

When you incur parental responsibility, and thereby the responsibility to love your child, it seems to be *your* love that is required since it is those parentally responsible for the child, and not just anybody, who are obligated to love the child. That *relational* obligation entails standing in a particular emotional relation toward another, and I'm not sure how that can be passed to someone else. To me, "Here, you love this baby" sounds like "Now that you are in a wheelchair, I don't love you anymore, but my friend Sally is willing to." The fact that the transfer is intended in advance, in the case of gamete donation, does not help. An intended violation of obligation is, if anything, worse than an unintended one. If children need the love of those parentally responsible for them and parental responsibility includes providing children with what they need, it may be impossible to transfer parental responsibility.

a) *What About Adoption?* We all know that parental responsibility is frequently transferred via adoption, an arrangement that is socially accepted. Acceptance of adoption may lead some to think that parental responsibility is easily and unproblematically transferrable. But the reasons for accepting a transfer of parental responsibility in adoption cases may not apply to other sorts of parent-child situations, including gamete donation or sale. Moreover, some may have accepted adoption too quickly or too simply, failing to realize that adoption is an inherently problematic arrangement, even if it is also often the best that can be done in a particular situation. Transferring parental responsibility via adoption may not be as simple as some may think, and it may not be relevantly similar to gamete donation.

There are some important differences between adoption and gamete donation, in addition to the current differences between the two in screening standards (high for adoption, nonexistent for gamete purchase) and payment to the biological parent (given to gamete sellers but not to parents relinquishing children for adoption). First, adoption is usually an ex post facto solution to the pressing problem of children whose parents cannot or will not care for them. The child is already there, and something must be done to care for her as best we can. This may differ, morally, from conceiving a child with the intention of transferring one's parental responsibilities, and for that express purpose, as a sperm donor does. If some parental responsibilities are of the emotionally relational category, and therefore not easily transferred, it may behoove one to take care not to incur those responsibilities unless one has a reasonable expectation of being able to fulfill them oneself. A sperm donor has deliberately done the opposite; a person relinquishing her child for adoption most often has not. Second, although parents who relinquish their children for adoption may claim to do so as an expression of their love for a child whose care they cannot undertake, it is hard to see how gamete donation can be an expression of love. "I loved you so much that I released you to a family more capable of caring for you," a parent who has relinquished a child for adoption may say to her biological child. But what comparable statement can a gamete donor make? "I loved you so much that I donated (or sold) the gamete from which you grew to someone else"? In what sense is that an expression of love, and who is the subject of that love? These differences give us pause in considering the analogy between adoption and gamete donation. Finally, adoption transfers parental responsibility from those who have it to those who did not (until they accepted the transfer), but sperm donation can sometimes "transfer" parental responsibility solely to the mother, who already has that responsibility. Can she meaningfully be said to now have more of it? If not, it is difficult to understand the sense in which the responsibility has been transferred rather than abandoned.

Even if we assume, incorrectly, that adoption and gamete donation are analogous, what conclusions should we draw from this (inaccurate) analogy? We can either decide that they are both unproblematic transfers of responsibility or that they are both problematic transfers of responsibility. I think they are both problematic. Adoption is not an ideal arrangement, even though it is often the best one can do in a difficult situation and may often turn out quite happily for all concerned. It is not uncommon for adoptees to wonder why their natural parents relinquished them for adoption and to struggle with identity, self-esteem, and feelings of rejection.[33] It is also not uncommon for biological parents to have persistent negative feelings about having relinquished their child for adoption.[34] That may be why it is commonly and accurately assumed that cavalier reasons for releasing a child for adoption indicate too cavalier an attitude toward one's parental responsibilities.[35] Adoption seems to be an attempt to make the best of a less than ideal situation. It is not itself an argument in favor of the unproblematic transfer of parental responsibility.

33. See David Brodzinsky, *The Psychology of Adoption*, Oxford University Press, 1990; Adele Jones, "Issues Relevant to Therapy with Adoptees," *Psychotherapy: Theory, Research, Practice, Training* 1997 34: 64–68; and S. L. Nickman, A. Rosenfeld et al., "Children in Adoptive Families: Overview and Update," *Journal of the American Academy of Child and Adolescent Psychiatry* 2005 44: 987–995.

34. See Jeffrey Haugaard, Amy Schustack, et al., "Birth Mothers Who Voluntarily Relinquish Infants for Adoption," *Adoption Quarterly* 1998 2: 89–97; and Maxine Weinreb and Bianca Murphy, "The Birth Mother," *Women and Therapy* 1988 7: 23–36.

35. Attitudes toward adoption likely vary by culture, but I would venture to guess that the need for parental love and unease at having been released for adoption are likely nearly universal. Similarly, I'd be surprised if the pain of not being able to raise one's biological child was a mere cultural artifact. These issues remain open to further findings.

b) *Can We Delegate Parental Responsibility?* We may think that while parental responsibility requires us to see to it that our child has a long-term loving relationship with a caregiver, we don't actually have to be that caregiver. Just as we may delegate our responsibility to shovel the snow in front of our house to a teenager in need of some pocket money, we may think we can delegate parental responsibility to others. But whether a responsibility can be delegated or not depends on whether it is a responsibility that different people perform in very different ways. It doesn't matter who brings the napkins for the birthday cake, but it can matter who bakes the cake. If you have teaching responsibilities, that requires you to teach, not to see to it that the class is taught. Responsibility to do things that different people do quite differently, such as teaching, singing, conducting, and, yes, parenting, seem to commit you to doing the job yourself (so long as you are able, of course). This doesn't mean that you can't hire a babysitter or a teacher, because those roles are not parental and leave the parental relationship intact. Hiring a nanny and sending your child to school are ways of fulfilling your parental responsibilities, not ways of delegating them entirely.

V CONCLUSION

Parental responsibility arises from our ownership and control over our hazardous gametes and belongs to those who own and control the gametes, so long as those gametes are not forcibly taken from them. Parental responsibility is probably not transferrable unless one is incapable of fulfilling it. Thus, the Hazmat Theory generates a high degree of nontransferrable responsibility to almost all of us at some point (since nearly almost all of us, at some point, are in possession and control of our gametes).

This may seem demanding and may leave us feeling weighed down by a serious burden. Yet some ways of thinking about pro-creativity would lighten this load considerably. For instance, if life is usually worth living for most people, maybe its worthwhileness will outweigh most of the difficulties our children will encounter, including the difficulty of having been created by irresponsible parents. If that is the case, why worry about the fine points of pa-rental responsibility and how it is incurred? If it is easily fulfilled, it is no great burden and we need not worry very much about incur-ring it. This view, which—sorry—is a huge mistake, may be in-ferred from the non-identity problem (another huge mistake), to which I will now turn.

Chapter 3

Is Procreation (Almost) Always Right?

I   THE NON-IDENTITY PROBLEM

Let us assume that some lives are worth living. If a life is likely to be worth living, it seems that it may also be worth starting, and permissible to create. A life worth living, by definition, is no worse than not living at all. Let us further assume, taking a sunnier view of life than might be warranted, that a child born to a fourteen-year-old mother will likely have a life worth living, despite a rough start. Parfit famously asks us to assume this and then asks: how can we persuade a fourteen-year-old girl to delay motherhood for her child's sake? *That* particular child will not be born if the fourteen-year-old delays pregnancy because a child born later will develop from different sperm and egg cells—she will be a *different* child. The teenager will have done the child she would have had at fourteen no favor.[1] If you are the person that grew from the particular combination of sperm and egg cells that combine to begin to form you, your window of opportunity for existence is incredibly small. Even minor changes to the timeline of events are likely to result in a different sperm cell fertilizing

1. See Derek Parfit, *Reasons and Persons*, Oxford University Press, 1984, Chapter 16.

that month's egg cell, so it turns out that almost anything we do affects the identity of future people. Actions take time; policies affect where people live, whom they meet, and whether, with whom, and when they procreate. Therefore, nearly everything we do and nearly every policy we enact affects future identities, especially since sperm cells don't live for very long. Given the millions of sperm in each ejaculation, even the time it takes to smoke a cigarette before rather than after intercourse will likely result in a different sperm fertilizing that month's egg and, consequently, the birth of a child different from the child that would have been born had you been more traditional and smoked after sex rather than before. Similarly, when a society considers whether to bury its hazardous waste in ways more or less conducive to the safety of future people, or whether to conserve or deplete natural resources, we may wonder who is harmed by riskier waste disposal or greater rather than lesser depletion policies since these policies affect the timeline of events such that enacting a different policy would result in the birth of different people.[2] So long as the policies we enact are still likely to result in people with lives worth living, we seem to be doing these people no harm, and therefore no wrong, by depleting resources or burying our hazardous waste less carefully since this is the best we can do for *them*. If we conserved more or disposed of our hazardous waste more responsibly, a different set of people would live with those results. So why not have a baby at fourteen, if you please, as you waste resources and bury your hazardous waste sloppily? These actions seem to harm no future person, so long as the extent of the suffering you

2. As explained in Chapter 1, policies affect things such as where people work and live, whom they meet, and thus if and when they procreate. By affecting if, when, and with whom people procreate, many policies and practices affect identities (by affecting which, of the many possible people, become future people).

cause by your selfishness will not result in people with lives not worth living. Who is your profligacy bad for?

The difficulty of identifying a person harmed or wronged by seemingly negligent procreative acts or policies has come to be known as the *non-identity problem*. The difficulty arises from the fact that the people who seem to be harmed or wronged by these seemingly negligent procreative acts or policies have lives worth living and would not exist at all in the absence of the acts or policies in question. It seems counterintuitive to say that teen parenthood does not harm the child born to a teen parent, but so long as these children have lives worth living, we seem to be forced to admit that teen parenthood was not bad for them. In fact, it was the very best their parents could have done *for them*. Better parents would have been someone else's parents (aren't they always?).

(i) The Non-Identity Principle The procreative principle that follows from the non-identity problem is: So long as our actions or policies are not likely to result in future people with lives that are not worth living, they are permissible (because they do not harm anyone). The non-identity principle would deem all procreativity permissible so long as the future person's life is likely to be worth living, even by the narrowest of margins. The non-identity principle is a narrow person-affecting principle because it judges permissibility on the basis of an act's or policy's effect on a particular, identified person. Ethical theories or principles that determine wrongdoing on the basis of how an act affects specific, identifiable individuals are narrow person-affecting theories. (For act x, we look at how x affects person p, q, r, and so on, to see whether x is permissible.) Wide person-affecting theories or principles judge permissibility of an act on the basis of its impact on people

in general, regardless of particular identities. (For act x, we look at the impact of x on the population or society that will live with the results of x.)

Some may think that if we cannot solve the non-identity problem, then we are stuck with the non-identity principle as our action-guiding procreative moral principle. That is not the case. If we can't solve the non-identity problem, we are only at risk of being stuck with the non-identity principle if we choose to stick with narrow person-affecting moral principles. So the problem is not nearly as pressing as some may think. In any case, we will solve the problem. In fact, we will dissolve it completely. It is not really a problem. It is a mistake.

I will begin by showing that the non-identity problem is a metaphysical mistake rather than a problem. The metaphysical mistake is the counting of existence itself as a good credited to its various causal agents instead of as a prerequisite for being subject to goods or to having interests, and a prerequisite that no real person can lack, at that. If we don't make this mistake, we don't generate the non-identity problem and thus have no need to solve it. However, if you are not convinced that I have dissolved the non-identity problem in the first half of this chapter, I will solve it for you in the second half. I will explain how deontological ethical theories, which are not narrow person-affecting theories, can point to the victim of procreative negligence and thereby solve the non-identity problem. Finally, even if we don't dissolve or solve the non-identity problem, we can easily avoid it. The way to avoid the non-identity problem is to adopt any ethical theory or principle that is not a narrow person-affecting one. Luckily, that includes all of the predominant ethical theories in modern philosophy. I will explain how we can steer clear of the non-identity problem by adopting any wide person-affecting ethical theory or any impersonal ethical theory.

There is no shortage of procreative problems but the non-identity problem is not one of them. The so-called non-identity problem is not a problem, and even if it were, it can be easily solved and even more easily avoided.

II DISSOLVING THE NON-IDENTITY PROBLEM

The non-identity problem is based on the idea that if something is good for you, so too, ultimately, is anything you need in order to get it.[3] If you need to take a bus to pick up your $1,000,000 lottery winnings, taking the bus is not bad for you even if it is a long, hot, stuffy ride. Sure, it's an uncomfortable ride, but if it's the only way for you to get your million dollars, it is not contrary to your interests to sweat it out. Similarly, if the only way to enjoy a life worth living is to be born to a fourteen-year-old mother, having a teen mother is not, all told, contrary to your interests. It would be better if you could have a mature mother, but you can't. It is not an option for *you*. If you didn't have a teen mother, you would never exist at all.[4]

You wouldn't exist at all. So what? Who needs to exist? No one. Nonexistence is no deprivation because there is no (real) person who lacks it. If you don't take the uncomfortable bus ride, you lose the lottery money, but if you don't exist, there is no *you* to lose, gain, benefit from, or be deprived of anything. No one is walking around looking for her lost existence, bemoaning the fact that she doesn't

---

3. I originally made a form of this argument in "Identifying and Dissolving the Non-identity Problem," *Philosophical Studies* 2008 137: 3–18.

4. Never existing at all is your "otherwise" condition in this case for purposes of counterfactual analysis of harm. Had your mother not had you at fourteen, you would never have existed (neutral value).

exist, or hanging out in some imaginary no man's land between existence and nonexistence, pining to enter into the golden realm of existence. We all exist. Woo hoo. Not only do you have no need to exist, existence is pretty much the only option for you. Sure, had your mother or father had a headache or a cup of coffee instead of conceiving you exactly when they did, you wouldn't exist, but *you* wouldn't *not* exist either. Never existing is not a real option for any real person. Therefore it does not seem to make much sense to count existence as a good that can offset or counterbalance some of life's burdens. Existence per se is neither a benefit nor a burden; it is a prerequisite for having interests, but it itself is not one of the interests that any (real) person has.

The mistake that generates the non-identity problem is the counting of existence itself as a benefit bequeathed to you by your ancestors and capable of offsetting life's burdens (either directly or by enabling you to enjoy life's benefits). Once we stop doing that, we have dissolved the non-identity problem. If we don't treat existence (per se) as a good capable of offsetting life's burdens, then the fourteen-year-old mother, for example, cannot use the fact that, but for her procreating at fourteen, her child would not exist at all, as a good that offsets or outweighs the burdens incurred by having a teen parent. We simply don't have a non-identity problem.

The fourteen-year-old mother burdens her child with all of the disadvantages associated with having a teenage mother. Those disadvantages may be mitigated (but not enough to make having a teen parent a good thing, all told) by whatever benefits there may be to having a teen mother, for example, by how energetically the teen mother plays with her toddler, but they are not mitigated or offset by the benefit of existence itself. Existence itself is not a benefit. Some things benefit us, some things burden us, but existing per se is just what it means to be a possible subject of benefits and burdens.[5] And no matter how delighted you are to find yourself eligible as a subject of benefits and burdens, that eligibility is not a gift or benefit bestowed upon you by your parents because it is something you didn't need and could not fail to have had.[6] Never existing is not an option for any real person because all real people exist. Even if you love life, if your ancestors bury their hazardous waste sloppily and you suffer from the ensuing pollution, that suffering is harm they inflicted on you (i.e., they have set your welfare interests back).[7] The fact that had they not done so you would not enjoy other life goods, such as, say, beer, is of no relevance because burying waste sloppily does not produce beer or provide beer-drinking opportunities. The only link between the beer and the sloppy waste burial is existence itself, which can provide beer-drinking opportunities but which you cannot fail to have. To continue our prior analogy, if your ancestors bury their waste sloppily, they have given you a ticket on an uncomfortable bus ride to the pub (where you will enjoy some rocking beer). Other people are riding on air-conditioned buses

5. I say a possible subject of benefits and burdens rather than simply a subject of benefits and burdens because most people think that some existing things, like rocks and dust, cannot be benefited or burdened. So while nothing has interests unless it exists, it may be possible for something to exist and still not have any interests.

6. Some might be tempted to think they almost "missed out" on existence. But if you never existed, you would not really "miss out" on anything. If you never existed, you would not really miss existing, nor would you really miss out on it because there would be no real you to miss or miss out on anythng. (Real FOMO—fear of missing out—is only for real people.)

7. I use harm fairly standardly, to mean "set welfare interests back." This is consistent with a counterfactual analysis of harm in which an act harms someone if it makes her worse off than she would have otherwise been. (In non-identity cases, we assume that had the act in question not occurred, the person in question would otherwise not exist.) It is also consistent with noncomparative analyses of harm (see Jeff McMahan, "Wrongful Life: Paradoxes in the Morality of Causing People to Exist," in *Rational Commitment and Social Justice*, Jules L. Coleman and Christopher W. Morris, Eds., Cambridge University Press, 1998, 208–248 and Jeff McMahan, "Problems of Population Theory," *Ethics* 1981 92: 104–107).

to the pub—no one has no way to get to the pub (i.e., everyone exists).[8] Your ancestors have harmed you with their sloppiness. They have made you worse off than you would otherwise have been. How? By polluting your environment. A polluted environment is bad for you (negative value). Never existing is not (neutral value).[9] Negative value is worse for you than neutral value. The beer and other life goods you enjoy (positive value) are not caused by or related to the polluted environment and are not credited to the polluters unless you are making the mistake of crediting them for your very existence, as a prerequisite for your life goods, thereby mistakenly crediting the polluters with the beer they never gave you and the opportunity to enjoy it that you could not lack.

When you assess your life, you can imagine a balance scale: on the good side, we put the beer, the chocolate, the friendships, and whatever other life goods you enjoy; on the bad side, we put the bad environment caused by the sloppy waste disposal, the allergies, the emphysema, the hunger, the heartbreak, and whatever other life badness you suffer. The bad stuff is bad for you and harms you. Some of that bad stuff is due to the environmental conditions caused by the sloppy waste burial. That harms you and it

8. It is true that if not for the sloppy waste burial, you would not be on any bus to any pub at all. But that would not be in any way bad or sad for you. "You" would just have turned out to be a merely possible person. And none of us, not even you—the real you, that is—have any reason to care about merely possible people. They are not sad to have no ride to the pub because *they do not exist* (and it is impossible for a nonexistent merely hypothetical entity to really be sad).

9. Not everyone accepts that existence has neutral value. Some think that since nonexistence is nothing, we cannot make any value judgments about it at all. But assigning nonexistence a neutral value is consistent with a "zero" or "nothing" value: neither negative nor positive. Those who reject comparisons between the value of existence and nonexistence regardless can reject the reasoning that leads to the non-identity problem since the non-identity problem relies on the view that a life worth living is no worse than nonexistence, which, in turn, implies a value comparison between existence and nonexistence.

is a bad thing in your life that you suffer from because your ancestors were sloppy. Their sloppiness harmed you. Simple as that. If the great friendships you have, say, are so great as to outweigh the bad stuff in your life, such that your life is worth living on balance, that does not make the bad stuff in your life any less bad for you, and it does not mean that the people who caused some of that bad stuff in your life did not harm you by causing that bad stuff. Your sloppy ancestors gave you emphysema, not friendship. (Granted, you would not have the great friendships had your ancestors not caused you emphysema because then you would not exist at all, but that would not be bad for you, nor is it a real choice for you.) Your fourteen-year-old mother did not give you "a life worth living," all told. What she gave you is a life with a fourteen-year-old mother. Your life, your existence itself, is like the scale—of neutral value. Having a fourteen-year-old mother is on the bad side of the scale. If you manage to secure many life goods, those goods will weigh heavily on the good side of the scale and outweigh the stuff on the bad side. If you don't manage to secure many life goods, then having a fourteen-year-old mother will weigh down the bad side of the scale enough to outweigh the stuff on the good side. But in either case, having a fourteen-year-old mother is bad for you and puts lots of extra weight on the bad side of your scale. By having you at fourteen, your mother has loaded up the bad side of your existence scale. That is bad for you and harms you. *The fact that had she not done so you would not exist at all just means that had she not done so we would not be balancing anything on any scale.* It does not somehow render the bad stuff on the scale an overall good, nor does it give your mother the right to credit for unrelated good stuff on the scale.

The mistake the non-identity problem makes is to put existence itself on the "good" side of the scale and credit it to your sloppy ancestors, either directly or by using your existence itself as a reason to credit the good stuff on the scale to your sloppy ancestors who did not provide that good stuff. Existence itself is not a good; it is just part of what it means to be subject to goods. It's like the scale itself, not like something on either side of a good/bad scale. The non-identity problem puts the scale *on* the scale, so to speak, and on its good side.

I will now elaborate on some of the significant points in the above argument in order to explain in greater detail just how the non-identity problem uses existence itself (and not life goods) to outweigh non-identity burdens and in order to further elucidate to whom our procreative concerns apply and how to properly conceive of future people.

(i) Does the Non-Identity Problem Use Existence Itself or Just Garden-Variety Life Goods to Justify Non-Identity Burdens? You might think that it is not existence itself that justifies non-identity burdens, but, instead, life goods—the beer, the chocolate, and so on. But, in fact, it is existence itself, and not just life goods, that does the justificatory work of supposedly outweighing life burdens in non-identity cases. The simplest way to see this is to note that sloppy waste disposal degrades the environment but does not contribute to beer production or provide beer-drinking opportunities. If your ancestors dispose of their waste sloppily and thereby trash your environment, that sets your welfare interests back. The fact that you can sometimes distract yourself from the bad environment by drinking some excellent beer is fortunate, but your sloppy ancestors cannot use that beer to excuse their sloppiness since their sloppiness has nothing to do with your enjoying that beer. "But you couldn't enjoy beer if you didn't exist and you wouldn't exist had your ancestors not

disposed of their waste so sloppily," you might argue. Sure. But notice that you just put existence back on the scale. You are only able to connect your ancestors' sloppiness to your beer enjoyment by crediting them with the existence that is a prerequisite for your beer enjoyment. (If you don't exist, it's really hard to drink.) It is thus your existence itself that is being used to justify your ancestors' sloppy waste disposal. Without giving your sloppy ancestors credit for your existence itself, you cannot justify their sloppiness. But, as argued, existence is not a good and therefore should not be credited to your sloppy ancestors. So we are left with the fact that your sloppy ancestors harmed you by trashing your environment.

Here's another example that helps clarify this point: Imagine that if any woman drinks significantly—say, four drinks a day—for six months prior to pregnancy (rather than during pregnancy, as is actually the case) her future child is likely to have a learning disability. Further imagine that Winey does this anyway because she likes her champagne. Her learning-disabled child, Cheery, enjoys existence anyway, especially chocolate, which her aunt gives her regularly. Arguably, the chocolate outweighs the learning disability. No mention of existence at all. Existence seems to have been kept off the scale. But now we have no connection between Winey's drinking and Cheery's chocolate. Winey's drinking harms Cheery by causing her learning disability, and Cheery's aunt benefits Cheery by giving her chocolate. We don't have a non-identity problem. We only generate the problem by putting existence back on the scale with the claim that had Winey not had the champagne, Cheery would not exist and would not be able to enjoy her chocolate-filled existence. When both benefits and harms are weighed against each other, chocolate may outweigh a learning disability, but one is still harmed by a learning disability unless existence is included in the equation, or placed on the scale. But since existence is not a benefit, is not needed, and cannot be lacked by any real person, it should not be used to outweigh or excuse any real person's real-life burdens. It has no business being *on* the scale; it *is* the scale.[10]

10. Still not convinced? Contrast the Winey case with that of Twinny, who uses fertility drugs to get pregnant, knowing it will make it likely that she will bear twins. Twinny gets pregnant and has twins. Her twins enjoy the companionship of twinhood but get annoyed sometimes by having a same-age sibling. Overall, though, they like being twins. But still, they challenge Twinny to justify her taking fertility drugs that she knew would increase the chances of them being twins and finding some features of twinhood burdensome. Twinny can explain that they like being twins, overall, and twinhood has both good and bad features. Since the good outweighs the bad and the goods and bads of twinhood are essentially and inextricably connected, they aren't harmed by being twins. If we weigh the goods and bads of twinhood, the goods of twinhood outweigh the bads for Twinny's twins. But this reasoning does not apply to a learning disability and chocolate (or to beer and a trashed environment), which aren't essentially or inextricably connected. Winey's champagne drinking does not cause or confer Cheery's chocolate; its only connection to the chocolate is its indirect conferral of existence that, in turn, provides the opportunity for the chocolate. Existence itself is the (alleged) benefit here. It is illegitimately weighing down the good side of the scale. The only reason that Cheery can't have chocolate without suffering from a learning disability is because she wouldn't exist if Winey had not taken the time to drink champagne prior to conceiving her; and if she didn't exist, there goes the chocolate. As we all know, learning disabilities don't cause or confer chocolate and neither does drinking champagne. Cheery, however, cannot have chocolate without a learning disability because she can only have chocolate if she has *existence*, which, in her case, comes along with a learning disability. Twinhood is itself bound to certain benefits and burdens, but a learning disability is not, in and of itself, bound to chocolate. For Cheery, it is only existence that binds her learning disability to her chocolate. Thus, it is existence that is being used to outweigh Cheery's learning disability. One might still argue that although existence provides Cheery's opportunity to enjoy chocolate, her learning disability is causally necessary for her existence and, therefore, causally necessary for her chocolate too. On this view, the learning disability is causally necessary for the chocolate, which outweighs its badness; again, no mention of existence at all. Except that existence is mentioned: it is invoked by discussing what is causally necessary for it, as if existence itself is a good that can justify the bad things that we need to endure in order to attain goods for which it is a prerequisite.

It is also worth noting that Cheery's learning disability per se is not necessarily causally necessary for her chocolate, nor is her mother's champagne drinking. Rather, innumerable circumstances are necessary in order for Cheery to enjoy chocolate, one of which (the champagne drinking) also happens to have caused Cheery to have been born with a learning disability. If Winey's drink of choice was orange juice, it would still have been causally necessary for Cheery's chocolate. Thus, it appears that orange juice could have facilitated

(ii) Possible, Actual, and Merely Possible People Let's take a step back to one hundred years before you were conceived. At this point, your existence is *possible*: it could happen or not. If it will happen, then you will exist and are, prior to your conception, what we might call a *future person*. You will exist, and those who exist already should care about you just as they care about themselves and each other. If "you" will never be conceived, then "you" are not and never will be a real person. Instead, "you" are a *merely possible person*, that is, a hypothetically possible union of gametes that could unite and grow into a person but never will. We have no reason to care about merely possible people[11] because they are not real and, therefore, they have no real interests.[12]

Cheery's chocolate-enjoyment opportunities without any associated learning disability. The learning disability can ride causally free of Cheery's chocolate. It may be a mere side effect of what is really causally necessary for Cheery's chocolate: the *time* it takes to drink the drinks, be it champagne that causes learning disabilities in future children or orange juice that only nourishes. The time it takes to drink the drinks provides for Cheery's opportunity to exist, and existence provides her opportunity for chocolate. If the drinks happen to cause a learning disability, it is existence itself that is used to counterfactually justify it: had Winey not downed the champagne that caused the learning disability, Cheery wouldn't *exist*, and one must *exist* in order to enjoy chocolate. Existence is doing the justificatory work here. It is its illicit weight on the scale that is outweighing the learning disability, and not the chocolate that can be there under many different circumstances. (Just so long as existence is there too ... —See? You can't run the non-identity calculation without putting existence on the life benefit-burden scale.) It is existence itself that is used to outweigh, and thereby supposedly justify, life burdens in non-identity cases.

11. Although some have regarded Parfit as claiming that a merely possible person can have interests and merit moral consideration, Parfit explicitly disavowed concern for merely possible people (in conversation and correspondence with me, years ago). Although one can infer such concern from Parfit's earlier work in *Reasons and Persons*, he did not intend to imply it. Parfit later deliberately distanced himself from such views, such that this view cannot be inferred from Parfit's discussion of the non-identity problem in his later work (*On What Matters*, Oxford University Press, 2011).

12. I make no claims here about possible persons in possible worlds. Maybe possible persons merit moral consideration in possible worlds, but "they" have no rights, interests, or actuality in the actual world. My views here are confined to the actual world.

a) *Future People Will Exist:* Although they do not exist now, all future people will exist (in the future), and all current people were once future people. If you are a future person, then you will exist. That is not fatalism or magic talk. It is just what it means to be a future person. If you exist now and enjoy your life, then ten years from now you may no longer enjoy your life. Your life may have become unenjoyable, or you may have become depressed and therefore unable to enjoy what would otherwise be an enjoyable life. We don't know which will turn out to be the case. It depends on how future events unfold. No fatalism, no magic, no metaphysical weirdness. But if you exist now, one thing we do know about you is that before you existed, you were a future person. How do we know this? Because that is what the term *future person* refers to: it refers to each and every person that will exist in the future. If you exist in the present but did not exist at some point in the past, then at some point prior to your existence you were a future person. If at some point in the past, instead of conceiving you, your parents got divorced and never saw each other again, then you were never a future person. "You" were a merely possible person, a hypothetical, merely possible entity that could have but did not turn out ever to exist.[13] Still no fatalism, no magic, no metaphysical weirdness.

---

13. In other words, your existence is not *necessary*. It's just that *if* you are a future person, *then* you will exist because that is true by virtue of what it means to be a future person. I am not saying anything like, "*x* exists now, therefore she was a future person one thousand years ago, and therefore her existence is necessary." Or, "Each future person is such that she must exist at some point; if that person is future person *x* then *x*'s existence is noncontingent and therefore *x* is a necessary being!" I am not making absurd metaphysical claims. I am making a simple claim about what is true by virtue of the meaning of the term "future person": "**If** *x* is a future person **then** *x* will exist." Thirty million years ago, you were a future person. If your mother had had a headache instead of a glass of wine forty weeks before you were born, then you might never have been conceived and you might never have existed. But that just means that if your mother had not conceived you, then thirty million years ago you were not a future person—you were a merely possible person, i.e., a hypothetically possible person that will never exist. The term "future people" picks out the people who will exist in the future.

So let's not be afraid to say what is true by definition: All future people will exist. We can then go on to say what is true by common sense: if all future people will exist, then it is reasonable for us to consider the existence of future people as a given, as something all future people come with, instead of as some special gift we give them. Interests begin with existence in place, providing us with a subject for interests.

b) *Epistemic Ignorance Is Not the Same Thing as Metaphysical Indeterminacy:* Let's take a step forward to one hundred years from now. In all likelihood, some people will exist. We are not sure who they will be. In other words, we don't know which of the possible people will turn out to be future people and which will turn out to be merely possible people. We should do the best we can with the knowledge we have to consider the interests of future people. We might decide to build all of our elevators with Braille pads listing floor numbers, in consideration of the interests of future blind people, even though it may turn out that future people have no use for these Braille pads because blindness will have become completely curable. In that sort of case, we might say that our epistemic limitations caused us to do something in consideration of the interests of future people that, as it turns out, doesn't do them any good. Similarly, if I save money for the second child I intend to have but never actually do have, I have erred in my consideration of the interests of future people because I was mistaken as to whom that category would include. But if, instead, I save money for the second child that I know very well I could possibly, but will not actually, have, then I am being foolish. I'm wasting my resources because I am setting them aside for a merely hypothetical entity that has no interests.

(iii) The Interests of Future People If you are a future person, you will exist. When you are born, you will have an interest in a robust set of procreative goods. Anything that anyone does that makes that set of goods smaller or weaker is acting contrary to your interests even if that act[14] is necessary for your existence. Why? Because you don't need to exist. What you need is *conditional* upon your existence so that *if* you exist, *then* it would be good for you to have a robust set of procreative goods. If we apply this reasoning to the non-identity problem, it is clear that procreative negligence harms the very people who suffer from this negligence. For example, let us imagine a conversation between the teenage mother, now middle-aged, and her child, now an adult. Let us also imagine that the adult child suffered the usual problems associated with having a teenage mother yet, through a combination of hard work, help from others, and good luck, he overcame some of these problems and has a life worth living as an adult:

ADULT CHILD: You harmed me by having me at fourteen.

MOTHER: I did no such thing. If I hadn't had you when I was fourteen, you wouldn't exist at all, and your existence is worthwhile, so I did not harm you by having you when I was fourteen.

ADULT CHILD: But I don't need to exist at all. Nonexistence would not be bad for me. Since I do exist, however, like most other people, it would have been good for me to have

---

14. Actually, it is not always the particular *act* that is necessary for your existence; sometimes it is only the *time* it takes to do that act. Sometimes, an alternate act that takes the same amount of time will have the same effect on the identity of who is conceived.

an adult mother, and it was harmful for me to have a teen mother. You harmed me by having me at fourteen.

MOTHER: You're right. Here I thought I could hide behind the non-identity problem but it turns out that the problem is not non-identity—it's me, having a baby at fourteen!

(iv) Puzzles of the Merely Possible By confining our concerns to real people and their real interests, we note that the non-identity problem does not arise because real people do not have an interest in existence itself and always have it anyway. However, if we confine our concern to future people and do not give any moral consideration to the hypothetical interests of merely possible people, we are left with some puzzling questions.

a) If Merely Possible People Don't Count, for Whose Sake Do We Refrain from Procreating the Miserable? Some may wonder whose interests we are thinking about when we decide not to create a child because her life would likely be utterly miserable.[15] We don't create her, so there is no actual person to point to as the object of our consideration. It can seem intuitive to say that we refrained from creating the utterly miserable person for the sake of the person that would have endured utter misery, had we proceeded with procreation. But we didn't proceed, so that person is neither a current nor a future person. She's a merely possible person: a hypothetically possible person that could possibly exist but will not. It can seem like we acted for her sake—for the sake of

---

15. I discuss this in greater depth in "Existence: Who Needs It? The Non-identity Problem and Merely Possible People," *Bioethics* 2013 27: 471–484.

a merely possible person. If merely possible people don't have interests and don't merit any moral consideration, why are we stopping ourselves from creating them, thereby moving them out of the merely possible category and into the future people category, if we so desire?

We stop ourselves because we don't want to put future people in positions of utter misery. We care about actual people and we don't want to do things that will make them utterly miserable. If we go ahead with the procreation in this case, we will have put a future person in a position of utter misery. That's why we don't: we refrain from doing something that would make a future person utterly miserable. Just as we don't make existing people utterly miserable (if we can help it) because we care about existing people, we don't create future people who are likely to be utterly miserable because, if we did, we will have made a future person utterly miserable. When we stop ourselves from making a promise we can't keep, it's easy to point to the person for whose sake we restrained ourselves—the person to whom we would have made the unkeepable promise. But when we stop ourselves from procreating a person whose life is likely to be utterly miserable, we can't point to the person for whose sake we restrained ourselves, but that's the reason we restrained ourselves. We exercised procreative restraint so that there would be fewer utterly miserable *real* future people to point to, not because we care about merely possible people.

Claiming that we restrained ourselves for the sake of the merely possible person we never created is senseless. If we want to go ahead and procreate the utterly miserable, why would we restrain ourselves for the sake of a merely possible person? That hypothetical entity doesn't even exist, so why would we put ourselves out for it? And if we are restraining ourselves for the sake of the merely possible person, then how come a future person suffers if we fail to restrain ourselves? That makes much less sense than what I argue here: when we restrain ourselves from creating the utterly miserable, we do so to avoid the creation of a *real* future miserable person. In other words, we restrain ourselves from creating the utterly miserable so that the set of future people will not include (or will include fewer) utterly miserable people. If we don't restrain ourselves, we will have done something terrible to a future person. Therefore, we restrain ourselves to avoid doing something terrible to a future person. I can see how this reasoning can seem like a bit of a parlor trick: we act for the sake of a future person and, in so doing, that person disappears in a "poof!" of retroactive non-existence. But the alternative explanation is even less sensible: we act for the sake of literally no one, for the sake of the "poof!" itself.

A much less confusing way to think about these kinds of cases is to consider them simply as cases where we refrain from doing something that would violate our principles, commitments, or duties. If act x would violate our principles, commitments, or duties, then we don't do it. Act x can be making a promise we can't keep or creating an utterly miserable person. These acts violate principles, commitments, or duties we have out of concern for real people and their real interests. (Just as we want there to be fewer real people experiencing the trust violation of a broken promise, we want there to be fewer real people experiencing utter misery.)

b) *If Merely Possible People Don't Have Interests, How Do We Excuse Our Creating a Miserable Person When Our Only Alternative Act Is to Create Another Equally Miserable Person?* Some argue that without appealing to the interests of merely possible people we have no way to deal with the following hypothetical moral dilemma:[16]

If we do *x*, we create miserable person *p*; if we do *y*, we create miserable person *q*.

What to do? Clearly, neither *x* nor *y*. If that is somehow impossible, then I think we have been put in a situation where we are forced to do something wrong. Because we have no choice, we are excused or not blameworthy. This is a case of a moral dilemma. There are various views about moral dilemmas: some think that there is no such thing as a moral dilemma, that is, there is always a permissible option; others, myself included, think that there is no reason to assume that you will never be confronted with a choice of two evils. You will then be forced to do something wrong but you are excused because you do not have a (right) choice. Procreation is not a special case regarding moral dilemmas: if you think moral dilemmas do not exist, you will think that it's okay to do either *x* or *y* because there is no more correct choice. If you think that moral dilemmas do exist, you will think that it is wrong to do *x* and also wrong to do *y* but you are excused from doing *x* or *y*, or not blameworthy, since you are stuck in a dilemma and don't have a (right) choice available to you.

If we must do either *x* or *y*, leading to the creation of either miserable *p* or miserable *q*, how does attending to the alleged interests of merely possible people help us? Some think that if we recognize that merely possible people have interests, then we can

16. See Caspar Hare, "Voices from Another World: Must We Respect the Interests of People Who Do Not, and Will Never, Exist?" *Ethics* 2007 117: 498–523. For a detailed response to these sorts of claims, see Rivka Weinberg, "Existence: Who Needs It?"

excuse our creation of p by appealing to the fact that had we not created miserable p, we would have had to create miserable q. Since miserable q never exists, the reasoning goes, we must be appealing to the suffering of the merely possible q to justify creating miserable p. But, it is argued, if we don't think that merely possible people have interests, then we cannot make this sort of appeal because q's suffering does not count since she is a merely possible person.

But, if creating miserable p is justified by the equally awful alternative act available to us (namely, the creation of miserable q), there is no need to appeal to the alleged interests of merely possible people to run this sort of justification: since we are responsible for the foreseeable results of our actions and to the foreseeable victims of our wrongdoings, if act x will result in a real, miserable person p, then this gives us reason to avoid act x, not because of the so-called interests of merely possible person p, but, instead, because if we do x, then a real person (real p) will suffer. So we should not do x, because, if we do, we will cause a real person (real p) to suffer, and we should not do y either because, if we do, we will cause a real person (real q) to suffer. When forced to do x or y, thereby creating (real) p or (real) q, we are excused from doing either one because we are stuck between a choice of two evils, or two wrong acts. There is no need to appeal to the interest of merely possible people in order to make sense of this case.

If we do make the mistake of attributing interests to merely possible people, we are led to comically counterintuitive results. Although we can't really do anything for the merely possible, we may act as if, so to speak, and set aside resources on their behalf— "the merely possible fund." Since there are innumerable merely possible people, the merely possible fund might have to be enormous. Setting aside even one penny for each merely possible person would bankrupt us and leave few resources for future people. Harming future people for the sake of merely hypothetical entities is wrong because it harms real people for the benefit of no one and for no morally respectable reason. It does not do very much for merely possible people either. In fact there is nothing we can do for "them" because there is no "them" to do anything for. If we understand the true metaphysical status of the merely possible, we will also understand the moral status that follows. A merely hypothetical entity that did not, does not, and will never exist cannot have any real interests, there being no real subject for said interests, and therefore does not merit any real moral consideration.

c) *Worse and Worse-r:* Another category of cases that may make some sympathetic to considering the hypothetical "interests" of merely possible people includes cases comparing procreative wrongs. One such case is Parfit's Ruth versus Jane example.[17] Ruth and Jane both have a genetic disease that will kill them painlessly at forty. Jane knows that her children will inherit the disease. She has a child anyway. Ruth knows that only her sons will inherit her disease and she can do prenatal genetic screening and in vitro fertilization to ensure that she has a healthy female child. She does not do IVF and has a diseased male child. We all think that Ruth did something worse than Jane. But why? They do the same thing (ignore risks to their future child) and cause the same outcome (create a baby boy that will die at forty). Is Ruth worse than Jane because she could have had a healthy child instead? That seems to implicate a merely possible person in our moral evaluation of the case. But we need

17. Parfit, *Reasons and Persons*, 375.

not do anything that metaphysically fancy to differentiate between Ruth and Jane and varying degrees of wrongness in cases
of this type. The reason that Ruth is morally more reprehensible
than Jane is because it would have cost Ruth less than it would
have cost Jane to avoid creating a child that would die at forty.
In order to avoid this outcome, Jane would have to refrain from
procreating entirely, but Ruth would just have to use technology
to select a female child. The less it costs you to avoid harming
someone or doing the wrong thing, the worse you are if you go
ahead and do it anyway.

We have now dissolved the non-identity problem and cleared
up some confusion about the morality and metaphysics of possible, merely possible, and future people. If you think some non-
identity residue remains, let us turn to a solution.

III   A DEONTOLOGICAL SOLUTION
TO THE NON-IDENTITY PROBLEM

A strangely overlooked fact about the non-identity problem is that
it does not apply to most ethical theories.[18] As we have noted, the
non-identity problem is aimed at narrow person-affecting theories,
that is, theories that hold an act to be right or wrong only insofar
as it affects a particular, identified individual. Virtue ethics focuses
on character development and the practice of virtue—clearly not
a narrow person-affecting ethical theory. Consequentialism determines the permissibility of an action based on its effects on the

---

18. This is particularly ironic because Parfit argues that the unacceptable implications of the
non-identity problem call for a new ethical theory entirely ("Theory x"). But none of the
central ethical theories we have on offer is subject to the non-identity problem since none
is a narrow person-affecting theory. See Parfit, *Reasons and Persons*, Chapter 18.

state of affairs. It is not a person-affecting ethical theory at all.[19] That leaves us with the third central ethical theory: deontology. Because the non-identity problem is often taken to apply particularly to deontological theories, I will take the time here to show that it does not. Deontology can solve the non-identity problem by pointing to the individual wronged, be the person harmed or not, by procreative negligence, and that person is the individual to whom others have been procreatively negligent (e.g., the child of the fourteen-year-old mother), regardless of whether her life is worth living.[20]

---

19. Although the non-identity problem is not aimed at consequentialist theories, consequentialism does not point to a victim harmed or wronged by non-identity type acts in many non-identity cases because, as noted, it is not a theory that determines wrongdoing on the basis of particular victim impact. Instead, it determines wrongdoing impersonally, on the basis of effects of acts on states of affairs. When the same number of people will be born, as in the case of a fourteen-year-old who can have a child when she is twenty-five instead, the state of affairs is better, from a consequentialist perspective, if she waits to conceive, but, in many non-identity cases, we do not have the same number of people born, and consequentialism can then run into non-identity types of difficulties. But it won't be due to non-identity reasons—meaning it won't be because we cannot identify a victim of procreative harm or negligence, since the existence of specific people who are made worse off as a result of an act is not needed for consequentialists to prohibit an act. Consequentialism requires maximization of the good of states of affairs. As such, it does not directly engage with the non-identity problem. Nevertheless, consequentialism does not seem to have adequate resources to deal with some non-identity cases; e.g., it cannot tell us why we should not create a much larger but much worse-off future population (so long as lives remain a net plus: worth living) rather than a smaller but better-off population, and it cannot tell us why we should not create a slave child who will be treated well enough so that her life will be worth living and may even result in a modest benefit to others. Consequentialism also runs into a related procreative moral difficulty, namely, Parfit's Repugnant Conclusion (see Parfit, *Reasons and Persons*, Chapter 17), which some might find even more problematic than the non-identity problem. For more on this topic, see Paul Hurley and Rivka Weinberg, "Whose Problem Is Non-Identity?" *Journal of Moral Philosophy*, forthcoming.

20. I originally made a more detailed form of this argument together with Paul Hurley in "Whose Problem Is Non-Identity?" Our argument extends and explains how the view that we can wrong people whether we harm them—i.e., set their welfare interests back—or not, works to solve the non-identity problem. The "wronging without harming" argument was made in various ways as a response to the non-identity problem but ran into difficulties

Deontological, or principle-based, ethical theories determine permissibility of an act on the basis of its conforming to a set of principles. These principles, usually Kantian in nature, are aimed at treating persons as having a special status that demands respect and constrains the ways they can be treated. Because Kantian theories focus on the status of each person as an end in themselves, they can be mistaken for narrow person-affecting theories because they are individualistic. Deontological theories do not permit sacrificing the individual for the sake of the group since they treat persons as ends in themselves, and not exchangeable in value. But they are not narrow person-*affecting* theories in the sense relevant to the non-identity problem because they do not determine wrongdoing on the basis of the *effect* of an act on an individual. They are not theories that determine permissibility of an act on the basis of consequences at all. Instead, deontological theories determine the permissibility of an act on the basis of its adherence to principles designed to treat people as having a special status as moral agents and ends in themselves. The non-identity problem does not apply to deontology because the non-identity problem is a problem only if permissibility of acts is determined by the act's *effects* or consequences on a particular person. Focusing on the effects or consequences of an act is a fundamentally nondeontological approach to ethics.

---

regarding arguments about consent, waiving rights, and how rights are determined. When we are clear about how deontology works, and the limits of the power of consent to waive rights away, it becomes clear that the non-identity problem does not apply to deontological theories. For earlier versions of "wronging without harming" arguments against the non-identity problem, see James Woodward, "The Non-Identity Problem," *Ethics* 1986 96: 804–831 and "Reply to Parfit's 'Comments on the Non-Identity Problem,'" *Ethics* 1987 97: 800–816; Parfit, "Comments on the Non-Identity Problem," *Ethics* 1986 96: 832–863; Gregory Kavka, "The Paradox of Future Individuals," *Philosophy and Public Affairs* 1982 11: 93–112; Parfit, "Future Generations, Further Problems," *Philosophy and Public Affairs* 1982 11: 113–172; and David Wasserman, "Non-identity Problem, Disability, and the Role Morality of Prospective Parents," *Ethics* 2005 116: 132–152.

(i) Clearing a Space for a Procreative Standard of Care Realizing that the non-identity problem does not apply to deontological ethical theories does not, by itself, tell us what our procreative duties are. It does not, by itself, set a standard of procreative care. It just clears up a confusion and provides us with a space to set the standard of care. Once we set a procreative standard of care, based on our deontological theories of persons and their rights, any act that falls short of that standard is a negligent wrongful act, regardless of its effects. And any person who is the subject of that negligent act is a particular person wronged by that act.

Because I view procreativity as an act that exposes future people to the risks of life, I think we should set the standard of procreative care in the same way that we set the standard of care for other activities we engage in which expose others to risks, as I explain in Chapter 2 and will set out in Chapter 5. Those who have a different conception of procreativity may have a different way of setting the standard of procreative care. The non-identity problem (and the non-identity principle that follows from it) has served as a constraint on the procreative standard of care because it implies that we don't harm anyone by creating her so long as her life is worth living and it (incorrectly) assumes that where there's no harm, there's no foul (or no wrong). The non-identity principle sets the standard of procreative care at a likelihood of a life worth living, overall. That is a very low standard. When we solve or avoid the non-identity problem, as we do in this chapter, we are free to set our procreative standards based on standard moral principles, which are likely to demand a higher standard of procreative care. In Chapter 5, I explain and defend my procreative standard of care, but in this chapter I free us of the non-identity constraint on our procreative standard of care. This freedom does not dictate a standard of procreative care. It just removes the non-identity constraint on whichever standard of procreative care we find fitting to set. Regardless of how we set the standard of procreative care and what that standard turns out to require of us, once we have a standard of care, any act that doesn't meet that standard is a negligent act, and any person subject to that act is a particular person wronged by that act.

Deontological theories grant rights to protect the status of persons as autonomous, as moral agents, as self-originating sources of claims, as deserving of respect for their own sake, and as interest-bearers. I will not expound on this at length here. For our purposes, it is enough to note some examples of deontological principles and see how they might apply to procreatively questionable acts, set a standard of procreative care, and solve the non-identity problem. I will then address Parfit's objections to resorting to deontology, or rights, to solve the non-identity problem. But first, a classic and a contemporary example of deontological theory and how each easily solves the non-identity problem.[21]

a) *Kantian Principles:* Kant's categorical imperative tells us to act only according to principles that it would be rational for us to will everyone to follow.[22] (This is Kant's famous requirement of universalizability.) Would it be rational for us to will everyone to follow the non-identity principle, which tells us that any procreative act is

---

21. We could go through more examples, but two will suffice to make the point because deontological theories are not subject to the non-identity problem since deontology does not evaluate acts on the basis of their effects (be those effects on individuals or on states of affairs). Deontological theories will solve the non-identity problem by pointing to the particular subject of procreative negligence as the person wronged by that negligence.
22. Kant, *Groundwork of the Metaphysics of Morals.*

permissible so long as the future person's life is likely to be worth living, even by the narrowest of margins? I don't see why it would be rational for anyone to endorse that principle when one could choose a procreative principle that generated a higher standard of procreative respect and care. Why would I want my ancestors to have abided by the non-identity principle? So that I can have a fourteen-year-old mother and a trashed environment? So that I can be a fourteen-year-old mother and trash the environment myself? If I endorse a principle that allows people to trash the environment, there may not be any environment left for me to trash, which violates Kant's requirement of universalizability. (Any principle that permits the trashing of the environment to the point that it leaves those living in it with lives just barely worth living risks unsustainability and is therefore not universalizable.) If I endorse a principle that permits adolescent procreation, I may die before I get the chance to procreate as an adolescent since having an adolescent parent significantly increases my chances of dying in infancy.[23] This poses a challenge to that principle's universalizability.

Similarly, endorsing the non-identity principle is not consistent with the Kantian value of treating persons as ends in themselves, with projects of their own to pursue. A life barely worth living is often a life with little freedom to choose and pursue one's ends. Acting in accordance with the Kantian requirement to treat persons as ends in themselves and never as mere means points us in the direction of a principle that sets a procreative standard of care

23. See Maureen G. Phipps, Maryfran Sowers, et al., "The Risk for Infant Mortality among Adolescent Childbearing Groups," *Journal of Women's Health* 2002 11: 889–897; and P. O. Olausson, S. Cnattingius, et al., "Teenage Pregnancies and the Risk of Late Fetal Death and Infant Mortality," *British Journal of Obstetrics and Gynaecology* 1999 106: 116–121; among many others.

that directs people to procreate when they are mature and to maintain a reasonably clean environment for future generations. That is clearly more respectful of people as ends in themselves, with their own purposes and projects to pursue, than the non-identity alternative, no? Which would you pick? Which do you think is more respectful of you as an end in yourself, with your own purposes and projects? I'd go with the principle that generates adult mothers and a reasonably clean environment, thank you very much.[24] Once we have that more stringent principle, any act that does not adhere to it is wrong, and any person subject to such an act has been wronged.

b) *Scanlonian Contractualist Principles:* Scanlon argues that if we take all persons to be of equal value and deserving of respect for their own sake, then we will act only in ways that others could not reasonably reject, as a principle of mutual governance.[25] Most people find it eminently reasonable to reject procreating as a teenager or burying hazardous waste sloppily.[26] Why would we choose the non-identity principle as a principle of mutual governance when we could set a higher, more protective standard of care that would be better for us? The fact that a different set of people will exist under one procreative principle rather than another does

---

24. Please do not tell me that I only say this because I am assuming that I will exist, regardless of which procreative principle is chosen—an assumption that violates the factual premises of the non-identity problem. I assume no such thing. What I assume, correctly, is that I will either exist, in which case I'd much prefer an adult mother, etc., or I won't exist, in which case nothing matters to me because I am a merely possible person—a hypothetical, nonexistent entity with no interests at all.

25. See T. M. Scanlon, *What We Owe To Each Other*, Harvard University Press, 1998, 106.

26. It is possible that disagreement over what counts as reasonable may make it difficult to set a Scanlonian standard of procreative care. But, to the extent that this is a problem, I take it to be a problematic feature of Scanlonian contractualism ("reasonable" can be deemed a response-dependent term, leaving room for much disagreement) rather than a problem with setting a deontological standard of procreative care, more generally.

not seem to argue in favor of a lower standard of procreative care. Here, too, we will set a standard of procreative care that is higher than the standard set by the non-identity problem. And any act that falls short of the higher standard will be wrong and wrong the person subject to it.

When we seek to abide by deontological ethics, we see that the non-identity problem is entirely beside the point.

(ii) Waiving Our Rights Goodbye? When Parfit initially considers the non-identity problem, he wonders whether an appeal to rights can solve the problem (by pointing to a victim of procreative negligence), but he concludes that it cannot because, he argues, we would waive our rights to, say, an adult mother, if having a teen mother were our only shot at a life worth living. Many early attempts to solve the non-identity problem by appealing to deontology ran into difficulties and rebuttals on these grounds.[27] When faced with rights-based solutions to the non-identity problem, Parfit argues that non-identity kinds of acts are not rights violations because, just as a surgeon can amputate an unconscious person's arm to save her life, relying on the patient's hypothetical consent to the unfortunate trade-off, the teen mother can rely on her child's hypothetical consent to the trade-off between a life worth living and the difficulties caused by having a teen mother.[28] Parfit argues that, given the choice, we would consent to the teen mother; we would not "rationally regret" having a teen mother, since that is causally necessary for the life worth living that we enjoy.[29] When we consider whether we would have consented to having a teen mother, or other forms

27. See note 12.
28. See Parfit, "Comments," 854–862.
29. See Parfit, *Reasons and Persons*, 364–366.

of what would otherwise be deemed procreative negligence in non-identity cases, we must consider two questions: First, would we consent to the procreative acts in non-identity cases? Second, if we would consent, would our (hypothetical) consent render the act permissible?

a) *Would We Consent?* The view that we would consent to the negligence necessary for our procreation evaluates the negligence from a first-personal welfare perspective and concludes that since we enjoy a life worth living, we would agree to the conditions necessary for that life that is, overall, worth living. I have already argued against this view by pointing out that procreative negligence harms the people who suffer from it so they should not consent to it. The fact that they otherwise would never exist is of no relevance since if they never existed, that would be just fine for "them," and, furthermore, never existing is not a real option for real people anyway.

Moreover, although whether an act is conducive to my well-being is certainly a factor I would consider when thinking about whether I would consent to an act, it is not the only factor. First-personal benefit is neither my only, nor necessarily my overriding, concern. I may care about how people are treating me regardless of the effects of their actions. If someone disrespects me or treats me like a tool for her own purposes, I might object to these actions even if they benefit me. For example, if my uncle gives me a new car, I would be delighted because I could sure use one, but if I later discover that he only gave it to me because he wanted to make his rebellious son jealous or impress his friends with his wealth, I might find his purposes or the fact that I am being used a mere tool for his purposes so objectionable that I would not consent to the act, even though it benefits me. Like most people, I care about myself first-personally, but I also have interpersonal, or what we might call second-personal, concerns.[30] I care about how people treat each other regardless of first or third-personal consequences. That is a deontological perspective, and it can resist non-identity reasoning because it does not grant ultimate or overriding value to first-personal benefit.

For example,[31] say I have a sexually transmitted disease that, if untreated, will be transmitted to anyone I have sex with and any children that might result from that activity. The disease is curable, but I choose not to take the medication to cure it now because it causes some temporary uncomfortable side effects. I figure I'll take the medication in a couple of months, when I have some time off work. Meanwhile, before taking the medication, I have sex, get pregnant, and infect my partner and my child. I have wronged them both by using them for my purposes and by caring more about my own temporary discomfort than theirs (the case is even worse if it causes birth defects or long-term damage to the child), thereby not treating them as moral equals and ends in themselves. I did the same thing to my child and my sexual partner (gave them a disease), and for the same reason (my own convenience). The fact that my child would not exist had I waited until I cured my illness does not render my wrong right, nor does it force my child to retroactively consent to my act. My act is wrong because it falls short of the procreative standard of care set by deontology, which, as argued, will be a standard far higher than the likelihood of a life-worth-living standard set by the non-identity principle. My child can find my actions objectionable enough on second-personal

30. Darwall calls these kinds of concerns second-personal, and he argues that it is this second-personal standpoint that is the basis for deontological ethics. See Stephen Darwall, *The Second-Person Standpoint: Morality, Respect, and Accountability*, Harvard University Press, 2009.

31. I owe this example to Paul Hurley. See Hurley and Weinberg, "Whose Problem Is Non-Identity?"

grounds to withhold consent, regardless of the on-balance, first-personal consequences.

Just as I object to my uncle giving me a car to make his son feel bad, I can object to my ancestors having buried their hazardous waste sloppily. It is not respectful of others to bury your hazardous waste so sloppily as to cause environmental damage because that falls below the standard of procreative care set by deontology and is therefore negligent. In acting negligently, you are not treating your victims as moral equals to you or as ends in themselves. The fact those who suffer from your sloppiness would not exist but for that sloppiness does not render your disrespectful treatment of them somehow respectful. It does not eliminate their grounds for objecting or not consenting to your actions because their objections are based on the way you treated them (negligently) and not on the overall first-personal consequences of that treatment.

b) *Does Consent Render Wrongs Right?* Even if I would consent to an act, that does not always mean that the act is morally permissible. The deontological requirement to treat persons as ends in themselves is part of a view of persons as rational agents, capable of setting their own ends. Therefore, it seems reasonable to think that when a rational autonomous agent consents to an act, that act does not disrespect the agent or treat her as a mere means. That's why one way to test for disrespect is to consider whether the person has agreed or would agree to the act in question. Consent can sometimes serve as an indicator of respect or disrespect. But not always.[32] Consent is not a reliable or appropriate indicator

---

32. For an excellent discussion of the relationship between consent and respect, see Arthur Ripstein, *Force and Freedom*, Harvard University Press, 71 and Chapter 5. For a discussion of the limits of consent, see Onora O'Neal, "Between Consenting Adults," *Philosophy and Public Affairs* 1985 14: 252–277.

of respect or wrongdoing when we are dealing with compromised agency or compromised ability to exercise rational agency due to extreme circumstances or vulnerability. These conditions occur frequently and are commonly cited as reasons for ignoring the presence of consent as a legitimizing factor.

Rational competence is often compromised in the very young, the very old, the naïve, the gullible, the less astute, and the emotionally or mentally unstable. When otherwise or partially rational agents are in these sorts of states, they are particularly susceptible to consenting to acts or arrangements to which they would, when or if more rational, refuse consent. That's why we find that people in these states are far more likely to fall prey to ill-conceived loans, inadvisable personal relationships, and imprudent purchases than their more rationally competent friends. Even the generally rationally competent among us can have their rationality clouded by greed, longing, rage, humiliation, jealousy, or fantasy, leading them to buy things or do things that they later not only regret but, in retrospect, can't believe they "fell for" or "fell into." (The "fall" refers to the fall from rational competence.)

Because our grip on rationality is so imperfect, we try to protect ourselves from our more dangerous imperfections. We don't just throw up our hands and say, "Well, we agreed!" Consent does not exhaust respect: when agency is compromised, as it so often is, rather than sanction exploitative conduct, consent or no consent, we try to enact safeguards against irrationality. We force ourselves to be more rational—we guard against agreements rendered suspect due to compromised or imperfect agency—usually by removing the irrational choice from our hands or by enacting laws against taking advantage of the irrationality of others.

Even when our rational capacities are functioning well, sometime we are driven to desperate "choices" by extremely difficult external circumstances such as poverty, disease, natural disasters, shortages, and so on. When we are truly desperate, we may feel compelled to agree to almost anything that promises to relieve our desperation. We might sell a kidney or steal money to buy one; we may agree to sweatshop labor conditions and wages. We might overpay considerably for a suddenly and temporarily valuable resource (e.g., batteries in a blackout). We may even sell our beloved children into indentured servitude. This is what vulnerability can do to us. It can render us blind with need, fear, or shame. It makes us ripe candidates for exploitation and blackmail. But when we yield to exploitation or blackmail, we are not operating as free agents participating in a shared or chosen end. Instead, we feel (and are) exploited, coerced, disrespected.

As a society, we do not happily accept choices made under conditions that render people too vulnerable to effectively exercise their rational capacity for appropriate, respectful self-governance. Rather than relying on the consent present in these kinds of cases, we recognize the consent as invalid or irrelevant, and we enact laws against transactions that are exploitative, since exploitation is not made right by the presence of consent.[33] We ban the sale of human organs, outlaw price gouging, forbid blackmail, set a minimum wage, and so on. We guard against our vulnerability to external circumstances by making it more difficult for people to take unfair advantage of another's hardship.

---

33. Cases in which the presence of consent does not render what would otherwise be wrongful rightful include, of course, consent under duress, cases where external circumstances render consent irrelevant, and cases where one is taking advantage of circumstances in an exploitative way.

This doesn't mean that any choice made in a desperate situation is invalid or irrational or should be disregarded. It just means that when consent is given, in desperation, to an act that would otherwise be deemed wrong, the mere presence of consent does not tell us that no wrong has been done.[34]

This is where Parfit seems to have a blind spot (or two). He assumes that consent is the same thing as respect, and he further assumes that if something does not make us first-personally worse off, then we have no reason not to consent to it and no reason to rationally regret it. In his discussion of the non-identity problem, Parfit argues that when we can't get someone's consent to an act, we should ask whether they could later rationally regret that act. He further argues that since the child of the fourteen-year-old mother or the people living in bad environmental conditions due to their ancestors' sloppy burial of hazardous waste have lives worth living, they cannot rationally regret their ancestors' acts because those acts did not make them (first-personally) worse off.[35] But these are both misunderstandings of deontology. Consent is not an exhaustive indication or test for respect, and we can have rational grounds for regret or for withholding consent or objecting to an act that does not harm us first-personally or harm anyone third-personally. We may have, as discussed, second-personal reasons for objecting to acts.

34. Sometimes the fact that the person agreed to being disrespected makes the disrespect even more objectionable and degrading because we now have two people disrespecting the victim: the perpetrator and the victim herself (think prostitution or eating bugs on TV so that you can star in a "reality" show).

35. See Parfit, *Reasons and Persons*, 373. In his later work, Parfit reiterates his understanding of the Kantian respect requirement as a requirement not to treat people in ways to which they could not rationally consent. He then restricts grounds for withholding rational consent to first-personal and third-personal effects on well-being, leaving out second-personal concerns entirely even though that is the locus of Kantian and deontological concerns. See Parfit, *On What Matters*, 1:181 and 186.

c) *Hypothetical Consent:* Although actual consent can sometimes justify an act that would be wrong in the absence of consent, like my entering your home (trespasser vs. guest), hypothetical consent is much more complicated and is less useful as a complete justification of an act. With regards to the non-identity problem, the kind of consent relied on by procreators and policymakers is hypothetical. It's easy to think of cases where hypothetical consent does not justify an act, even one that would be justified by actual consent. If you're away on vacation and unreachable, I can't redecorate your living room to suit what I know to be your taste, even if you would have agreed had you been asked. Even cases that seem to rely on hypothetical consent for their legitimacy, such as my breaking into your cabin in the woods to save my life during a blizzard, probably don't rely on hypothetical consent alone for justification. I think it would be okay for me to break into your cabin in the woods to save my life during a blizzard even if you left a sign on the door saying, "Don't Come In! Not Even to Save Your Life During a Blizzard!" Something other than just your hypothetical consent justifies my breaking into your cabin here. The limited justificatory power of hypothetical consent further serves to undermine "consent" as an objection to the deontological solution to the non-identity problem.

IV   IMPERSONAL OR WIDE WAYS AROUND THE NON-IDENTITY PROBLEM

Because the non-identity problem is a problem for narrow person-affecting theories, it can be avoided by wide person-affecting theories as well as non-person-affecting theories. There are many wide ways around a narrow problem and many impersonal ways around a person-affecting problem. Often people think they are "solving" the non-identity problem when all they are doing is forging another wide path around it.[36] Solving the non-identity problem can only be done by pointing to the victim of procreative negligence. Avoiding the non-identity problem can be done by adopting any nonnarrow person-affecting ethical theory. (As a nonnarrow person-affecting ethical theory and as a theory that is able to point to the victim of procreative negligence, deontology both solves and avoids the non-identity problem.) By avoiding the non-identity problem, we avoid the non-identity principle as well and are free to set a procreative standard of care higher than the low "life worth living" non-identity problem standard, but we don't thereby solve the problem. Instead, we steer clear of it. The advantage to solving the problem is, of course, that it is then solved. The advantage to steering clear of the problem is that we have no need to solve the problem. In this chapter, I have explained how we can do both: We have metaphysical reasons to dissolve the problem completely (allowing us to point to the particular victim of procreative negligence as we would normally do, without non-identity worries). We have a deontological way to solve the problem by pointing to a particular victim of procreative negligence. And we can steer clear of the problem by adopting any ethical theory that is not narrowly person-affecting.[37]

---

36. Examples include Hare, "Voices from Another World" and Elizabeth Harman, "Can We Harm and Benefit in Creating?" *Philosophical Perspectives* 2004 18: 89–109, among others.

37. Another option is to accept the non-identity problem. Although most find its implications disturbing and counterintuitive, some simply accept it with no further discussion or analysis, which is somewhat mystifying. David Boonin, however, argues that accepting the non-identity problem is not as counterintuitive or as morally disturbing as one might think. See Boonin, *The Non-identity Problem and the Ethics of Future People*, Oxford University Press, 2014.

It is time to stop being mesmerized by the non-identity problem. The resources we have to deal with it have been vastly underestimated.

Once we break the spell cast by non-identity reasoning, we are forced to consider our procreative responsibilities more seriously. Actually, even if the non-identity problem remained in full force, it would still not excuse procreative negligence. It would remain a problem to be solved, not a blanket excuse for procreative misconduct. We burden our descendants in many ways and harm them with all the difficulties we inflict on them. Life is difficult, at many points and in many ways, for almost everyone. So why do we keep making more people go through it? Are we obligated to stop? That is the question I address in the next chapter.

Chapter 4

Is Procreation (Almost) Always Wrong?

Some people think that life is bad. I am one of those people. I think that life is, on the whole, and in most of its parts, bad. Irredeemably bad. Even when it's good, it's bad. Other people, probably most people, think that life is good. Even when it's bad, it's good. I should say that the optimists have a different but equally valid perspective. I think that is the reasonable conclusion. But I can't get myself to really believe it. Instead, my intuition that the optimists are blind, deluded, and wrong persists. If my gut is right, having children is probably almost always wrong because, if life is bad, then we are putting people into a bad situation by creating them. (I say almost because there may be cases where the interests in procreating may be strong enough to outweigh the interests of future people for whom it would have been better, on the pessimistic view, never to have been born.) The case for this view has been forcefully made by David Benatar.[1] I will begin by discussing this dark view. I will

1. See David Benatar, *Better Never to Have Been: The Harm of Coming into Existence*, Oxford University Press, 2006. Benatar also presents an argument based on the alleged asymmetry between pleasure and pain; i.e., the absence of pain is good even if it is not enjoyed by anyone but the absence of pleasure is not bad if it is not suffered by anyone. I have argued against Benatar's asymmetry elsewhere and will not focus on it here, as I don't consider it to be his strongest argument for the conclusion that coming into existence is a harm. It is a "best explanation" argument: Benatar argues that his asymmetry best explains four other common

then consider whether having children is always wrong even if life is usually, on balance, good for those who live it. After all, we don't ask children if they would like to be born. Seana Shiffrin argues that procreation involves a problematic consent rights violation.[2] I will consider whether this argument is persuasive. I will then assess, overall, whether having children is always wrong and show that although neither of the central lines of argument for that conclusion succeeds, we are left with some worries that may not be fully resolvable.

I IS HUMAN LIFE, OBJECTIVELY, BAD? IS IT AN OBJECTIVELY BAD EXPERIENCE AND OF LOW QUALITY?

(i) Kinds of Value Benatar argues that life is bad and bad for those condemned to live it. When he says life is bad, he means that it is a bad experience for people and that most or even all people live lives of low quality in terms of well-being. That is what I mean as well when I say that life is bad. It's a bad experience and of low quality in terms of well-being. Experiential value is one sort of value. Well-being and the quality of life are one measure of life's value. There are many other sorts of value and ways of valuing

---

beliefs. But not only are there simpler and more intuitive explanations of those beliefs, it is far from clear that the four beliefs up for explanation are actually widely held to be intuitive, and it is even further from clear that Benatar's asymmetry is not more counterintuitive than the beliefs are intuitive. (So, if forced to accept Benatar's asymmetry or abandon the four beliefs it is alleged to best explain, it seems likely that many, if not most, would choose to abandon the four beliefs.) For a refutation of Benatar's asymmetry argument, see Rivka Weinberg, "Is Having Children Always Wrong?" *South African Journal of Philosophy* 2012 31: 26–37. I argue against Benatar's view that life is bad for people and therefore having children is wrong in that paper as well, but I develop that argument further here.

2. Seana Shiffrin, "Wrongful Life, Procreative Responsibility, and the Significance of Harm," *Legal Theory* 1999 5: 117–148.

human life: moral, aesthetic, scientific, and so on. What we are concerned with here is life's experiential value and human well-being. If life's a bad trip, we shouldn't send people on it. That's the pessimistic view I'm talking about.

This is separate from questions regarding the moral value of existing persons. We may hold, with Kant, that all persons have intrinsic moral worth due to their rational capacity for moral agency. This worth demands our respect and places constraints on how we may treat people. For example, it entails that we may not treat persons as mere means to our own ends. This view, by itself, does not tell us very much about the experiential value or quality of human life. We may think that all life is sacred and valuable morally, spiritually, or even aesthetically, but again, that is a different kind of value from the kind we are now considering. It may be that these other ways of deeming human life valuable (or not) are important enough to override concerns about the experiential value of life for people and human well-being, but, on most accounts, that will not be the case. Most nonexperiential and non-welfare accounts of the value of human life apply to those already in existence and do not provide an independent and overriding reason for creating new life regardless of how awful it will be to live it (in terms of experience and well-being). The kind of value we are concerned with here is the experiential value of human life and human well-being.

(ii) The Quality of Human Life (Well-Being) How to assess the quality of human life is something that no one has quite figured out, though not for lack of trying. Some look to simple hedonistic measures of pleasures and pains, others to the fulfillment of desires, or to objective lists of capabilities that contribute to a life of human flourishing. Benatar argues that life is of low quality on

all of these three accounts because we suffer way more than we acknowledge, we live in a state of many unfulfilled desires and adapt by not desiring the unattainable, and we don't really flourish at all if we expand our objective list of well-being by imagining what a really good life experience would be like.[3] This is a difficult set of views to prove.

On hedonistic measures, even if Benatar is correct in claiming that we discount the hunger that precedes our satisfaction of it,[4] pleasure and pain are to some degree inherently subjective measures. If we enjoy satisfying hunger, we may enjoy hunger due to anticipation of satisfying it, and then the fact that hunger precedes its satisfaction can be thought of as a win-win. Some take great pleasure in merely "being alive." It gives them great joy. From a baseline temperament like that, the hedonistic glass will nearly always look at least half-full. Insisting that it is really half-empty is not more objective. It is just a different interpretation and evaluation of the hedonistic value of experiences.

On desire-fulfillment measures, it is likely true that we modify our desires to what we think attainable because to do otherwise is painful and sometimes irrational, like crying for the moon.[5] That may be a good reason to reject this method of evaluating well-being, but, if we accept this method, then the fact that we modify our desires to those that we can fulfill will only help us fare well. The fact that a desire must gnaw at us, disturbingly, before we fill it is a pessimistic interpretation of desire. Others may see an

---

3. For Benatar's discussion of the experiential value and quality of well-being of human life, see Chapter 3 of *Better Never to Have Been*.

4. See Benatar, *Better Never to Have Been*.

5. See Amartya Sen, *Commodities and Capabilities*, Oxford University Press, 1985, 21 and Cass Sunstein, "Preferences and Politics," *Philosophy and Public Affairs* 1991 20: 3–34.

unfulfilled desire as an exciting time, filled with anticipation and enjoyable striving. It is far from clear that, "objectively," people fare poorly on desire-fulfillment measures of well-being.

On objective-list measures, it is hard to know what to make of Benatar's claim that human flourishing is pathetic compared with any kind of flourishing we could imagine,[6] for even if that is the case, it does not show that people fare poorly in objective terms. We may not fare as well as we would if we could fly, see many more colors, and understand way more than we seem to be able to, but that does not mean that people do not fare well on objective-list measures of the quality of human life in its actual rather than possible capabilities.

None of the above measures of the quality of human life is completely divorced from the way it feels to live (even the objective-list method includes many subjective elements like being able to experience happiness, pleasure, etc.). Ultimately, the subjectivity of our evaluation of the quality of human life, particularly our own, is where the crux of Benatar's argument lies: he argues that life doesn't really feel as good as we convince ourselves that it does and that we are deluded in our assessments of the experiential quality of our lives.

(iii) The Experiential Value of Human Life How does it feel to live a human life? What kind of an experience is it? Most people say, "Good!" Benatar argues that this is a mistake, that people tend to be deluded optimists. And he can explain why: we are evolutionarily adapted to think that life is better for us than it actually is; we are programmed to be Pollyannas. Of course, not all of us suffer from Pollyanna syndrome. I don't. But does that

---

6. Benatar, *Better Never to Have Been.*

make me a more objective evaluator of the quality of human life, or am I just suffering from Scrooge syndrome instead?

a) *Pollyanna or Scrooge? Pick Your "Syndrome":* Benatar argues that the world's many optimists suffer from a Pollyanna-type syndrome that makes them view the world through rose-colored distortive glasses and to embrace life as an adaptive preference: we are alive so we are motivated to like life, much as a woman in a sexist society has a motivation to prefer her own second-class status. She will have the second-class status anyway, so she might as well put a good spin on it. Benatar further argues that the rosy, distorted vision of life may be a result of natural selection since a more accurate assessment of life would likely decrease reproduction and increase the likelihood of suicide.[7]

Is life, *objectively*, bad? I can only claim, against my intuitive protest, that there is no way to know for certain since there is no objective perspective we can access in order to assess whether life is actually bad for people even though most of them seem to think it's good for them. And most people—with some quiet (depressed?), loud (philosophers? poets? rock stars?), or dead (by suicide) exceptions—seem to think that their lives are well worth living and that they are relatively happy and well off.[8] There are psychological studies that show that people generally tend to forget or ignore bad life experiences more than good ones, but this does not mean that this tendency blinds them to the reality

---

7. Benatar, *Better Never to Have Been*, 65–69.
8. See Ed Diener and Carol Diener, "Most People Are Happy," *Psychological Science* 1996 7: 181–185; David G. Meyers and Ed Diener, "The Pursuit of Happiness," *Scientific American* 1996 274: 70–72; Angus Campbell, Philip E. Converse, and Willard L. Rogers, *The Quality of American Life*, Russell Sage Foundation, 1976, 24–25; Margaret W. Matlin and David J. Stang, *The Pollyanna Principle: Selectivity in Language, Memory and Thought*, Schenkman, 1978, 146–147; among many others.

of their lives. It may just be a question of focus or a retrospective appreciation of the meaning or value that a difficult experience has given them. There is also research showing that depressed people generally have a somewhat more realistic view of their own abilities and future prospects.[9] But that research only shows that depressed people have a more realistic idea of themselves and their prospects. It does not show that they have a more realistic view of reality, generally, or of the human condition. Furthermore, some research seems to vindicate the common-sense view that people feel happy and think their lives are good when they live free from persecution and abject poverty.[10] This may indicate that so long as future people are not likely to suffer persecution or abject poverty, they are likely to enjoy their lives.

Just as being an incorrigible Scrooge does not show that life is good or bad for people, being resolutely optimistic, even in an unrealistic Pollyanna sort of way, does not prove that real life, without the rose-colored glasses, is objectively good or bad for people. The good in life could still balance out or outweigh the bad from a more objective perspective. But we will never know because we have no access to a more objective perspective from which to evaluate the value of human life, generally. It would be nice if, when evaluating the human condition and human life, we had more to go on than subjective, individual assessments. It may seem weak

9. See L. B. Alloy and L. Y. Abramson, "Judgment of Contingency in Depressed and Nondepressed Students: Sadder but Wiser?" *Journal of Experimental Psychology* 1979 108: 441–485; and K. Dobson and R. L. Franche, "A Conceptual and Empirical Review of the Depressive Realism Hypothesis," *Canadian Journal of Behavioural Science* 1989 21: 419–433.

10. Ed Diener et al., "Subjective Well-Being: Three Decades of Progress," *Psychological Bulletin* 1999 125: 276–302. Saul Smilansky cites Diener to make this point as part of his argument toward the conclusion that life is usually good and that people's positive assessments of their lives are usually reason based rather than illusory. See Smilansky, "Life Is Good," *South African Journal of Philosophy* 2012 31: 69–78.

to argue that life is good based on nothing more than the perspectives of individuals, yet which other perspective can we access? I am not arguing that all value is inherently subjective. It is important to remember that we are speaking here only of a certain kind of value, namely, the experiential value of human life and the quality of human well-being. I am arguing that the perspectives of ourselves and other people are the only ones available to us from which we can, in any meaningful way, evaluate the experiential value of human life and human well-being. There is no accessible objective view or evaluation of the experiential value of human life and well-being.

(iv) Is The Preference for Life an Adaptive Preference? Because we have no accessible objective perspective regarding the experiential value of life, the common individual preference for life is not analogous to standard adaptive preference cases in which, for example, an oppressed woman expresses a preference for her second-class sociopolitical status. Her perspective may be skewed by her lack of better and viable alternatives or by her ignorance of what her life could be like in a more egalitarian society. We, living outside of her sexist society, may be better positioned to understand this. Similarly, if someone is color-blind, she likely does not experience her deprivation and, therefore, may not feel a loss. But we who see in color know what the color-blind are missing. We know of their deprivation. Life, however, is a position we all occupy, so there seems no "outside" position from which to assess its value. Moreover, we are similarly stuck in the confines of the perspectives of ourselves and other people. (Who else can we hear from? The universe? The impartial spectator? God? Few, when appropriately medicated, have heard from these sources.)

Benatar suggests an error theory and provides an evolutionary explanation for it. According to this view, we are mistaken as to the quality of our lives because Pollyanna syndrome is adaptive. It discourages suicide and encourages reproduction. Maybe. But it may also be the case that we are not in error and thus in no need of an explanation of a nonexistent error. It is worth noting that there are evolutionarily adaptive explanations for anxiety, depression, and pessimism as well. Being a Scrooge is adaptive too. It makes us careful, more likely to anticipate, note, and avoid danger, and it also makes us more protective of our young, which enhances survival and reproductive success.[11] Just as we may deem optimists bedazzled Pollyannas, we may call pessimists myopic Scrooges. There is no objective way to settle this. We can only look at what people tend to think about their lives. And from the perspective of most people, life usually seems worth living despite its challenges. Sometimes, it is claimed to be worth living *because* of its challenges.

a) *Subjective Evaluations of Suffering:* In his 1999 Academy Award acceptance speech, the director Roberto Begnini enthusiastically and sincerely thanked his parents "for the greatest gift of all: *poverty!*" The actress Cate Blanchett, whose adored father died suddenly when she was ten, "has called bereavement 'a strange gift.' In many essential ways . . . her father's death was the shadow that informed her brightness. 'It's chiaroscuro,' she said."[12] Valuing

---

11. See Robert Leahy, "Pessimism and the Evolution of Negativity," *Journal of Cognitive Psychotherapy* 2002 16: 295–316; Matthew Keller and Randolph Nesse, "Is Low Mood an Adaptation? Evidence for Subtypes with Symptoms That Match Precipitants," *Journal of Affective Disorders* 2005 86: 27–35; and John Lehrer, "Depression's Upside," *New York Times*, February 28, 2010; among many others.

12. John Lahr, "The Disappearing Act," *New Yorker*, February 2, 2007.

one's suffering is not limited to actors in the film industry (we just hear from them the most because they get the most airtime). The psychologist Victor Frankl famously did not regret his excruciating experiences in the Nazi death camps because he felt that the experiences enriched his understanding and appreciation of the meaning of life.[13] One may think that, in these kinds of cases, it is the benefit derived from the painful experiences that is valued and not the pain or suffering itself, but that's not how the value is described by the people in the examples above. They describe the pain itself not as an unfortunate but necessary means to the benefit but as itself a benefit. A friend of mine who had been very depressed and lonely his entire adult life surprised me by saying, "I *love* life!" I laughed very hard at this and looked at him quizzically. He stared at me, shocked at my obtuseness, and said, "Yes, of course I'm unhappy right now but basically, I love life and have always loved life."

Of course, there is an alternate view of life. As H. L. Mencken said: "How little it takes to make life unbearable: a pebble in the shoe, a cockroach in the spaghetti, a woman's laugh." Misogyny aside, I "know" that Mencken is right. But I see no vantage point from which to argue that my view is "objectively," or in any authoritative sense, correct. We can all agree that life is treacherous and difficult, but many claim that suffering is outweighed by life's goods and can also be meaningful and valuable. I don't see how to settle the matter because there is no "overriding" or "more objective" perspective accessible to us in this kind of case. This is not a numbers game per se. It's not the fact that most people find life worthwhile that makes it so. Rather, my point is that among the different ways of interpreting experiences and evaluating life's

13. Victor Frankl, *Man's Search for Meaning*, Hogger and Stoughton, 1971.

quality, neither the optimistic nor the pessimistic is more authoritative or objective than the other. (However, if the vast majority of people found life awful or not worth living, that would, clearly, make it more difficult to claim that procreation is morally permissible.) We are forced to take people's views at face value and most people claim to experience and consider life meaningful, worthwhile, and good.

It seems that people tend to be constituted to value their lives. Does this apparent constitutional peculiarity make procreation not (almost) always wrong?

II   AN EXPERIMENT

Say we ran an experiment, to satisfy our curiosity about being creators, designed to create Peeps: sentient, conscious, intelligent, and self-conscious beings who have everyday, enjoyable, and even some unusually great experiences but who also suffer considerably in many ways. Many lead lives of great anguish. Peeps experience physical, mental, and emotional suffering, but they tend to enjoy many aspects of their suffering, or perceived goods that come along with or are derived from their suffering, either directly or interpretively (by attributing great meaning and value to them). If you ask them, as they wince from the pain, whether they are glad to exist, they answer, emphatically: "Of course!" If you point out to them the fact that they are wincing, they either say, "Sure, but in order to appreciate happiness, I need to know its opposite," or, "But other times I am dancing and laughing," or, "Yes, but wincing makes my life meaningful, fulfilling, and excellent." A small minority does not enjoy any aspects of their suffering at all. Some of them even kill themselves. Are we doing anything wrong by running this experiment? "Of course we are," say the pessimists. "We are making persons suffer and it is only adding insult to injury to make most of them masochistic or wired just weirdly enough to derive enjoyment from it."

But the optimists are not even clear on how or why we are asking the question. "What suffering?" they ask. "Enjoyment is not suffering. You have no basis for calling enjoyment and the experience of meaning suffering at all. If anything, we are doing the Peeps a favor by creating them. Look how much they enjoy and value their lives. Who are you to tell them that they don't or shouldn't enjoy and value their lives?"

I call this a draw, of sorts. In order to conclude that our experiment—which is, loosely, akin to what we might be doing when we create people—is permissible, the following conditions must apply:

(i) We Have to Have a Very Strong Interest in Running Our Experiment; in Other Words, in Procreation Otherwise, why run the risk of being wrong and causing great suffering for no equally important reason?[14] Remember our miserable minority. The fact that most Peeps (or people) love their existences does not, by itself, cancel out the sizable minority who don't. Merely

---

14. Some argue that our interest in procreation partly justifies the potential harm inflicted on future people, but their accounts of procreative justification tend to rely less on this interest than my account does here. John Robertson, for example, argues that procreative liberty justifies procreation, but he does not worry about procreative harm much because he accepts non-identity reasoning and the non-identity principle (see John Robertson, *Children of Choice: Freedom and the New Reproductive Technologies*, Princeton University Press, 1994, Chapter 2). David DeGrazia argues that procreative liberty justifies procreation but only partially. He argues that children have an interest in being born and this interest combines with the impersonal value of adding good to the world and procreative liberty to justify procreation in cases where it is reasonable to think that the future person will be happy (and not deludedly so) to have been born. (See David DeGrazia, *Creation Ethics: Reproduction, Genetics, and Quality of Life*, Oxford University Press, 2012.)

hypothetical Peeps (or people), who are not created, lose nothing and are deprived of nothing by not being created. It is far from clear that we can claim to be running the Peep experiment for Peeps' sake. Instead, we can admit that we are running the experiment (or procreating) for our own sake and that we have a strong and legitimate interest in doing it. That may help excuse us from the complaints the miserable minority may lodge against us. After all, we knowingly created them. (Though, presumably, we do not know which particular procreative act will result in a member of the miserable minority. If we do know that a particular procreative act will create a miserable person, it would seem that we have a strong reason not to proceed with procreation in that case.)

Because our interest in procreativity is crucial to its permissibility, the importance of procreative motivation is further underscored. Our interest in procreativity includes our reasons, or motivations, for procreating. If our reasons were manipulative, cruel, or disrespectful, say, then our interest in procreating would be objectionable on those grounds, and less capable of serving as a ground for permission to procreate. Thus, we have further confirmation of the importance of paying attention to procreative motivation.

(ii) We Have to Mitigate Damages Since we knowingly risk creating miserable Peeps (or people), we must try to mitigate the damage we cause by trying to limit the size of our miserable minority, perhaps by improving our ability to assess which ways of running the experiment or which instances of procreativity are more likely to result in miserable Peeps (or people). We must also try to help them deal with their predicament. (Can't they just kill themselves if they are not happy with life, and be done with it? More on that at the end of this chapter.)

(iii) We Must Be Confident That Life Is Not Objectively Bad If life is objectively bad and only seems good to those suffering from Pollyanna syndrome or a surfeit of serotonin, then it does seem hard to justify running the Peeps (or people) experiment. If life is really bad, we should probably stop perpetuating it. Alternatively, if we could be sure that life is good for people (in terms of its experiential quality and human well-being), then procreation would not be (almost) always wrong. It might even be right. If it is reasonable for people to believe that life is good but it turns out that life is actually bad, procreators will not be at fault since their acts will have been justified by their reasonable beliefs at the time. The worry about life's badness remains a moral worry, though, for those who think it is also reasonable to think that life is bad.

I conclude that it is only if we have a significant and nonobjectionable interest in procreating, are likely to be able and willing to mitigate some of the damage we cause if we turn out to have procreated the miserable, take pains to minimize our risks of procreating the miserable, and are confident that life is not actually bad, that we can hope to conclude that procreation is not (almost) always wrong. Many people, perhaps even most, are optimistic about meeting these conditions. They will have an easier time deeming procreation often permissible (even good!).[15] Those of us,

---

15. Some go so far as to deem procreation required. The argument for requiring procreation is usually based on existence or life being deemed good. If life is good, some say, more life is even better. Consequentialists tend to split regarding whether consequentialism requires making people happy or making happy people (see Jan Narveson, "Utilitarianism and New Generations," *Mind* 1967 76: 62–72 and "Moral Problems of Population," *Monist* 1973 57: 62–86). Others have argued that procreation adds value to the world and is something we may be required to do for others, in order to do our part to make the world a good or better place (see Saul Smilansky, "Is There a Moral Obligation to Have Children?" *Journal of*

myself included, who are less than fully confident that we can meet the aforementioned conditions, despite the fact that life seems so good to so many, must face the possibility that procreation may be (almost) always wrong.

III   IMPOSING A RISK

What of the miserable minority? They are a small minority as a percentage of the population, but they are still sizable. If our interest in procreating is strong enough, and the risk of procreating a miserable person is low enough, perhaps we can justify our risk imposition (just as we permit imposing other sorts of risks on others to further our interests so long as the interest is strong enough and the risk is low enough . . .). I will return to this question in Chapters 5 and 6, when considering procreating under various circumstances that have a significant likelihood of resulting in significant difficulties for future persons.

However, we may also wonder whether we have any right to be imposing any risks on future people at all. Existing people share the world with us, and our activities impose risks on each other, which we permit for the benefit of all. Banning all risk imposition would be practically impossible (merely breathing imposes risks of contagion on others). If we banned all risk imposition, life would quickly grind to a painful and abrupt halt for all of us. Thus, it makes sense for us to allow certain kinds of risks between us

---

Applied Philosophy 1995 12: 41–53). Since I have argued that no one has an interest in existence itself and since I think the claim that life is so good as to require us to produce more of it is unsupportable, even by Pollyanna standards (even Pollyanna must concede that *some* lives are awful and we can't always know in advance which ones will turn out to be the horrific ones), I will not pursue those arguments further here.

existent folk. But why drag new people into the risk pool? Ah, we are back to that. Because it's fun to swim, remember? It is *worth* the risk; it is a *reasonable* risk, in many, if not most, cases.

(i) Imposing Risks Without Consent Seana Shiffrin famously objects to this line of reasoning.[16] She argues that procreation involves the imposition of a huge risk for the sake of what she calls a "pure benefit,"[17] that is, something that is good but whose absence would not be considered a harm or a deprivation. Pure benefits, argues Shiffrin, can only be imposed on others if we have their actual consent. When we procreate, we cannot be said to have the future person's actual consent; therefore, argues Shiffrin, procreation is always morally problematic.

This argument relies on the intuition that we have different attitudes to harms and benefits: harms are important to avoid but benefits are not always important to secure; harms are more objective but the value of benefits is more subjective.[18] Given these differences between harms and benefits, Shiffrin argues that although we can rely on hypothetical consent when we impose a risk on people in order for them to avoid an even greater harm, if we impose a risk in order for them to obtain a "pure benefit," we must have actual consent.[19] Since procreation imposes the risks of life on a child for the sake of a "pure benefit," procreators would seem, on this view, to require their child's actual consent to being procreated. Of course, they cannot get their child's actual consent to being procreated. And therein lies the problem. There is no solution.

16. Shiffrin, "Wrongful Life."
17. Shiffrin, "Wrongful Life," 124–126.
18. Shiffrin, "Wrongful Life," 130–133.
19. Shiffrin, "Wrongful Life," 126.

Shiffrin illustrates her view with the following analogy:

Imagine a well-off character (Wealthy) who lives on an island. He is anxious for a project (whether because of boredom, self-interest, benevolence, or some combination of these). He decides to bestow some of his wealth upon his neighbors from an adjacent island. His neighbors are comfortably off, with more than an ample stock of resources. Still, they would be (purely) benefited by an influx of monetary wealth. Unfortunately, due to historical tensions between the islands' governments, Wealthy and his agents are not permitted to visit the neighboring island. They are also precluded (either by law or by physical circumstances) from communicating with the island's people. To implement his project, then, he crafts a hundred cubes of gold bullion, each worth $5 million. (The windy islands lack paper currency.) He flies his plane over the island and drops the cubes near passers-by. He takes care to avoid hitting people, but he knows there is an element of risk in his activity and that someone may get hurt. Everyone is a little stunned when this million-dollar manna lands at their feet. Most are delighted. One person (Unlucky), though, is hit by the falling cube. The impact breaks his arm. Had the cube missed him, it would have landed at someone else's feet.[20]

Shiffrin argues that Wealthy had no right to impose the risk of being hit by gold cubes on nonconsenting island inhabitants. He could—and probably would—take that sort of risk himself, but imposing it on someone else, argues Shiffrin, transforms

20. Shiffrin, "Wrongful Life," 127.

the broken arm into a wrongfully imposed harm rather than a voluntary cost. Conclusion: both Wealthy and every procreator commit morally problematic acts because they impose risks for the sake of pure benefits without the imposee's actual consent.[21] Imposing life on children, without their consent, is, says Shiffrin, "in tension with the foundational liberal, antipaternalistic principle that forbids the imposition of significant burdens and risk upon a person without the person's consent."[22] Thus, "One way to think about this view of procreation as morally problematic is to say that procreation violates the consent rights of the child who results."[23]

(ii) Children Do Not Have Consent Rights While Shiffrin's argument captures many a teenager's sentiment ("I never asked to be born!") and has intuitive appeal, it is not clear that it applies to procreation. Some may think it odd to entertain arguments based on the consent or lack of consent when speaking of as yet nonexistent beings, incapable of consent.[24] However, Shiffrin is not attributing consent rights or autonomy interests to merely possible people or to any nonexistent being. Her view is that procreation violates the consent rights of actual children, who are born without their consent. On this view, all real children are born into a

21. Shiffrin, "Wrongful Life," 129. Shiffrin notes that such acts may still be ultimately permissible, all things considered, though she does not specify the circumstances under which permissibility would pertain.
22. Shiffrin, "Wrongful Life," 137.
23. Shiffrin, "Wrongful Life," 137.
24. Recall, from Chapter 1, the claim that worrying about a future person's consent or lack thereof to her own existence may be thought of as a category mistake since consent does not apply to future beings. However, also recall the opposing view, which takes the fact that future people are incapable of consenting to their own existence to be a way of describing the concern about "forcing" someone into life rather than a factor that alleviates that concern.

state of violated rights. Taking this argument on its own terms,[25] we can note that the risks of life are imposed on (real) children and children do not have autonomy or consent rights because they aren't competent to exercise them. Children are incompetent: they require our paternalistic care, and paternalists are allowed—indeed, in some cases, they may be required—to impose risks on their charges for the sake of pure benefits. Competence is what differentiates procreation from the gold-dropping case. The island inhabitants are competent agents, so we cannot paternalistically impose on them, even for their own benefit. Children, in contrast, are not competent agents, and we may therefore legitimately assume paternalistic authority and impose risks upon them for their benefit, including for their "pure benefit." Children cannot grant legitimate consent because they are not competent to do so. Their consent is neither necessary nor possible.[26] Instead, paternalistic authority can be appropriately exercised over children. Our doing so does not violate liberalism's antipaternalistic principle because that principle doesn't forbid paternalism on behalf of children. Thus, it cannot be liberalism's antipaternalistic principle (which often forbids activity that affects others without their consent) that makes procreation always a problematic consent rights violation.[27]

---

25. One may object to taking the argument on its own terms and object to the analogy in ways having nothing to do with consent. For example, the people in Shiffrin's case suffer a bodily injury and receive a marginal benefit, especially given its disruptive effect. But I set these concerns aside here. Because I respond directly to Shiffrin's central claim, i.e., that procreation violates children's consent rights, my response has the virtue of speaking directly to the core of Shiffrin's general argument structure. My response does not preclude challenging Shiffrin on other grounds as well, of course.

26. I am not arguing that children will retroactively consent to their parents' procreativity. I am arguing that children do not have consent rights and therefore their consent to their own creation is not necessary.

27. Shiffrin, "Wrongful Life," 137–138.

a) *Objection: Children Grow Up:* It may seem as if we are getting away with something too quickly here—as if we are exploiting children's temporary incompetence to impose a series of lifelong risks (i.e., the risks that living a life entails) upon them. Procreation imposes life not only on children but on the adults they will become.[28] After all, one lives one's entire life, usually only a small portion of which is spent as a child. Assuming that human life typically begins in some embryonic stage, passes through birth and on into infancy, childhood, adulthood, old age, and then death, one may wonder why a procreator, who foreseeably imposes life on a person throughout all of those life stages, can claim to derive the right to do so based on the paternalistic authority that only exists during the earliest stages of life.

Reply: Paternalism is justified in cases of incompetence, for the duration of the state of incompetence, be that incompetence permanent or not.[29] The only difference that duration of incompetence makes to the justification of paternalistic acts is that when we have reason to believe that a person's incompetence is temporary, we should not make decisions for her that can be put off and made by the person herself once competence is regained. That's why we don't rearrange our friend's furniture while she is sleeping or sell her car for her while she is under anesthesia. But if our friend is in drug rehab and deemed temporarily

---

28. I thank Paul Hurley, Suzanne Obdurzalek, and Dion Scott-Kakures for helpful ideas and discussion regarding this objection.

29. Incompetence is not the only way to justify acting on another's behalf without the person's consent. Examples of cases where paternalism may be justified even though all the agents involved are competent include emergency situations when something important is at stake, cases where one has reason to think that the person would consent if asked, and situations where one cannot ask for consent. For example, if you step into the street as a car you don't notice is barreling toward you, I can yank you back out of the way of the oncoming car. What is important to the procreative case, though, is that children's incompetence justifies paternalism on their behalf.

incompetent, we might sell her car for her to pay for her continued care; if our friend is very drunk, we may hide her car keys for the night. Childhood is temporary, yet paternalism is justified during childhood nonetheless. Because procreation imposes life on children, paternalistic authority can explain why procreation does not violate future persons' consent rights despite the fact that the incompetence of childhood is not lifelong and despite the fact that life is.

The lifelong effects of procreative paternalistic decisions differ little from many other paternalistic decisions made on behalf of children (and other temporarily incompetent persons) that will have lifelong effects. Giving children violin lessons, choosing not to give children violin lessons, circumcision choices, dietary choices, educational choices, and so on, all have long-term effects. Paternalists are required to make decisions on behalf of their charges, including decisions that have long-term or lifelong effects: Violin lessons or the beach? Surgery, chemotherapy, or both? Cochlear implant or not? . . . Sometimes, if a decision can be postponed until competence is acquired or regained, it may behoove the paternalist to postpone the decision until the agent can competently make it for herself. Life, or the decision to be born, is not the kind of decision that can be postponed by the paternalist until the charge acquires or regains competence. Making that decision on behalf of one's charge may therefore be an appropriate exercise of paternalistic authority.

We may wonder whether the fact that we give birth to children rather than to adults capable of autonomy is a trivial, contingent fact that is not significant enough to rebut Shiffrin's argument. For if we gave birth to adults, who do have autonomy and consent rights, then Shiffrin's argument would be stronger because she could more successfully argue that competent adults are born into a state of consent rights violated. Unlike children, adults have the consent rights in question, providing a basis for a claim to their violation. It is, of course, quite difficult to imagine creating autonomous adults since an autonomous life seems to require experience and training, or at least some getting accustomed to the way the world is. But let's set that difficulty aside. We still find that, while the fact that we give birth to children is contingent, it is not trivial. A large part of the reason we want to have children is to experience the joy, meaning, and fulfillment of playing a paternalistic parental role in nurturing a child toward an autonomous adulthood. It is difficult to imagine what our motivation would be for creating autonomous adults.[30] Even companionship would not be guaranteed since an autonomous adult can choose her companions. Sustaining the earth's human population or creating a workforce to support us in our old age might motivate the procreation of autonomous adults, and I suspect that those motives

---

30. David Wasserman suggests a futuristic case: The environment is no longer suitable for children but we are able to create adults with adult cognitive capacities who, due to their inexperience, still need considerable adult guidance. Would it be objectionable, on consent grounds, to create these pseudo-adults? I am not sure that the creation of these pseudo-adults could be parentally motivated or otherwise acceptably motivated. I am also not sure that it would be fine to create people born into an environment that could not support children—I'd want to know more about what was deficient in the environment and how it might affect the newly born pseudo-adults. But, setting all of those considerations aside, I do think that a consent issue would come into play in this sort of case, provided that these pseudo-adults were sufficiently competent as to have consent and autonomy rights upon birth. Another case suggested by Wasserman is that of adults who deliberately create a child who will never attain competence. It may seem perverse that this couple is less susceptible to consent rights violation charges than adults who try to create a child that will eventually become competent. On my view, both couples are equally free of consent rights violations, as I argue above. The wrong that adults who deliberately create a child who will never attain competence do is to deliberately create a child so cognitively disabled as to never achieve competence. Their wrong is not that they violate (or don't violate) their child's consent rights.

would render procreation much more problematic (would we be using those adults as a mere means to our ends?). Shiffrin's argument would have far more force if procreation resulted in autonomous adults rather than in nonautonomous babies. But it doesn't, and that fact, although contingent, is not trivial. It is the fact that pushes open a gap between the unjustified paternalism in the gold-dropping case (because the island inhabitants are competent) and justified paternalism in procreative cases (because children are incompetent).

(iii) Imposing a Risk for the Sake of a Pure Benefit Paternalistic authority, however, does not justify any and all acts. Can paternalistic authority justify our imposing a risk for the sake of pure benefits (which is what we seem to be doing when we procreate)? And, if so, is it reasonable to deem life a pure benefit that is rationally worth its risks?

a) *Can We Impose Risks for Pure Benefits?* In cases of legitimate paternalism, we don't really have two agents at all. Instead, we have one agent who is responsible for making choices on behalf of her incompetent charge. Agents make choices that often involve trade-offs and risks. Just as it would be odd and unjustified to prohibit agents from taking risks for the sake of pure benefits for themselves, it is equally odd and unjustified to bar paternalistic agents from taking risks for the sake of pure benefits for their incompetent charges. That is part of what a paternalist is *supposed* to do. Paternalists are supposed to assess choices on behalf of their charges and make the choice that seems to be in their charges' best interests. Just as it can sometimes be in our own best interests to accept risks for the sake of pure benefits, it can sometimes be in the best interests of our charges for us to do so on their behalf.

Determining when this is the case and acting accordingly is part of a paternalist's job.

Our justified paternalism toward children requires us to make decisions that we would make for ourselves, including choices that involve weighing risk versus benefit, choices that involve more than one rational option, and choices that involve incurring risk or harm in order to obtain a pure benefit. We think nothing of teaching children or mentally incompetent adults to ride bicycles or ice skate, activities that risk harm for the sake of pure benefits. Similarly, it's permissible to take a demented person for an enjoyable walk in the park even though she might get congested from the pollen. These examples illustrate the fact that, when paternalism is justified, the caretaker appropriately and justifiably makes decisions on behalf of her charge that are, all things considered, in the interests of the charge. This includes decisions that involve risking or even definitely sustaining harm (who doesn't fall when learning to ride a bike?) in order to obtain a pure benefit. Paternalists are required to act in the interests of their charges, including obtaining pure benefits for them, even if this entails risking harm, so long as the risk is rational to impose for the sake of the benefit.[31] Is it?

b) *Betting Someone Else's Life: Is Life Worth Its Risks?* When acting paternalistically, we cannot use consent as our guide because our charges are not competent to provide it. Therefore, it may seem reasonable to guide our paternalistic activity by what our charge would be likely to consent to if they were competent, that is, by

---

31. There are various ways of assessing the rationality of a risk. One way is to consider whether the ideally informed rational agent would be likely to take the risk (for the sake of its likely benefits).

their hypothetical consent.[32] Or we can simply guide our paternalistic activity by the decisions that are most likely to be in the best interests of our charge.[33] Most often, these two kinds of guidelines for paternalists will point toward the same decision since informed, competent agents are likely to consent to that which furthers their interests. The point here is that when deciding on behalf of others, we generally ought to try to take reasonable risks and to guide our choices by what the person would want, were she competent, provided that we have some knowledge of the kinds of things the person would want (as in the case of, say, your elderly, incompetent mother, whom you know well). If we don't know what our charge would want, were she competent, we ought to do our best to make reasonable decisions and take rational risks, guiding ourselves by what most rational, informed people might want or at least by what is usually deemed reasonable by most informed competent agents.

Yet a degree of paternalistic conservativeness or caution may be in order.[34] It's one thing to decide to go bungee jumping yourself for the sheer thrill of it but another to dangle someone else's life from a rubber band. It may be okay to try to get to the top of Mt. Everest because it is, after all, there, but sending your thirteen-year-old kid on that trek is more questionable. On the other hand, to be an overly risk-averse paternalist is often seen as overprotective, and contrary to the interests of one's

32. See Ronald Dworkin, "Paternalism," *Monist* 1972 56: 64–84.
33. See Cass R. Sunstein and Richard H. Thaler, "Libertarian Paternalism Is Not an Oxymoron," *University of Chicago Law Review* 2003 70: 1159–1206.
34. Rawls relies on this view to justify veiling probabilities in the original position. He argues that since those in the original position are making choices on behalf of others (i.e., their descendants), they are required to be extremely cautious and risk averse. See John Rawls, *A Theory of Justice*, Harvard University Press, 1971, 168–170.

charge.[35] That thirteen-year-old shouldn't be climbing Mt. Everest, but if you don't let him walk around the block, you're not furthering his interests.

Finally, when it comes to children, it is often thought best to guide our paternalistic choices by what may usually be deemed reasonable by informed, competent agents, while also attempting not to foreclose a child's future autonomous choices unduly.[36] Some have gone so far as to claim that a child has a right to an "open future."[37] While it's unclear to me that anyone can have an open future (none of us can flap our wings and fly off into the sunset, and many choices close off alternative choices), since children are generally only in a state of temporary incompetence, taking care not to foreclose a child's future autonomous choices unduly or unnecessarily does seem warranted.

So, these, roughly, are our paternalism guidelines: act reasonably to further the interests of one's charge, erring slightly on the side of caution, and taking care not to foreclose future choices unduly. What do these guidelines tell us about procreative paternalistic activity?

Life is a high-stakes game that need not be played.[38] Not playing is clearly the more conservative, risk-averse choice. Yet, if playing is

35. Rawls has been widely criticized for being overly risk averse, and his claim that risk aversion is required when making decisions on behalf of others has not proven particularly persuasive. See Ronald Dworkin, "The Original Position," *University of Chicago Law Review* 1973 40: 500–533; R. M. Hare, "Rawls' Theory of Justice," in *Reading Rawls*, Norman Daniels, Ed., Stanford University Press, 1989, 81–107; and Thomas Nagel, "Rawls on Justice," *Philosophical Review* 1973 82: 220–234; among many others.

36. See Joel Feinberg, "The Child's Right to an Open Future," in *Whose Child? Children's Rights, Parental Authority, and State Power*, William Aiken and Hugh LaFollette, Eds., Littlefield, Adams, 1980, 124–153.

37. See Feinberg, "Child's Right."

38. Shiffrin lists four factors that contribute to the difficulty of relying on hypothetical consent for procreation: not procreating will not harm future people; procreation may cause future people severe harm; being created cannot be escaped without high cost; and the hypothetical consent is generic (Shiffrin, "Wrongful Life," 133). The first three of these difficulties speak to the nature of the risk procreation imposes but still do not show the risk to be irrational. The last of these difficulties is discussed above.

still, all things considered, rational and often quite rewarding, it is a risk permissible to impose, as a paternalist, on one's charge. Shiffrin argues that the hypothetical consent relied upon in procreative cases is generic and "not based on any features of the individual who will bear the imposed condition." This is taken to reduce the legitimacy of relying on hypothetical consent as a procreative guide. But the fact that the hypothetical consent relied upon in procreative cases is generic seems appropriate since we do not know what the future person will be like, but we may well bet that she will possess what I take to be an extremely peculiar feature shared by most people, namely, the love of life. Shiffrin highlights the fact that life is quite risky, but that does not mean that the risk is irrational to impose paternalistically on one's charge. So long as the risk is worth taking and not contrary to what the charge would likely competently choose (as discussed above), it is permissible for the paternalist to impose the risk on her charge.

Since most informed, competent agents seem to regard life as a reasonable risk, since life does not foreclose a child's future autonomous choices, and since life is usually deemed to be not contrary to the best interests of those who live, procreation does not appear to be always morally problematic by virtue of violating the future person's consent rights.

It may be argued that assuming consent to having been procreated based on the fact that most people seem happy to be alive or seem to deem their life eminently worthwhile (i.e., a valuable experience and of high quality) is not warranted. We do not know that the person we procreate will be glad of her life, nor do we know that human life is generally worthwhile, regardless of how humans seem to regard it.[39] To the first point, it seems

---

39. See Benatar, *Better Never to Have Been* and "Why It Is Better Never to Come into Existence," *American Philosophical Quarterly* 1997 34: 345–355.

reasonable for paternalists to rely on that to which most would reasonably consent, as is the case in all matters paternalistic in which specific preferences are not known. However, in order to claim that most would reasonably consent to life, we come up against the second point regarding the experiential value and well-being quality of human life, generally. It must be conceded that if human life is not worth living, then we ought not to procreate, but it also must be conceded, as we noted earlier, that it is difficult to claim that human life is not worthwhile regardless of how humans regard the worth of their lives. We are human, so we have no other vantage point from which to judge whether human life is a worthwhile experience. If it seems worthwhile to most of us (though I still don't understand why), it is hard to see how we can claim it not to be worthwhile for most of us. So, once again, we arrive at the conclusion that it is probably permissible to procreate persons whose lives are likely to be deemed worth living, especially by them.

c) *If Life Is Worth the Risk, Do We Have a (Paternalistic) Obligation to Create It?* If adults, as paternalists, can permissibly impose the risks of life on their children, does that imply that these adults are obligated to do so when the risks of life would appear to be worth taking, for those future children? No. Since all interests are contingent upon existence, we are never obligated to create a person for the sake of that person. However, if we want to create a person and it is otherwise permissible, we need not concern ourselves so much about violating that person's consent or autonomy rights since the person we will create will be a child and, as such, will not have these rights, as argued above.

(iv) Lingering Worries But these antinatalist arguments leave us with some lingering worries . . .

a) *The Experiment:* If we think back to our Peeps-creating experiment in terms of consent rights, it will be immediately obvious that no such experiment would ever pass an IRB (Institutional Review Board) assessment. We can't experiment on persons without their consent. That's basic. So why can we conduct our Peep or procreative experiment on children? Are they not persons?

Procreation, however, is disanalogous to the Peep experiment in a few important ways: First, as argued, procreation creates children, and children do not have consent rights. Parents have paternalistic authority over their children. Unlike the case of Peep creation, in the procreative case, parents consent on behalf of their future children to their children's creation. So we do have some sort of consent, be it the child's hypothetical consent or the parents' consent on their child's behalf. Children can be enrolled in scientific studies based on parental consent, and it is the same kind of paternalistic authority that we may rely on in the procreative case. The fact that the interests of prospective parents may conflict with the interests of their future children tells us that paternalism will not do as a stand-alone procreative guide. Paternalistic authority may show that procreation does not always involve a problematic consent rights violation, as I have argued, but it will not tell us everything we need to know about when procreation is permissible or impermissible. For that, we will need a theory that can adjudicate the conflicts that arise between prospective parents (who are interested in procreating) and future children (who are interested in a fantastic life). I will take this up in Chapter 5. Second, when permissibly procreating, our intent is not to use our children for experimental or other purely end-driven purposes. Rather, our intent is to engage in a mutually beneficial and respectful relationship with them. This makes our procreative enterprise less sinister seeming than the hypothetical Peep experiment, presumably conducted to satisfy human curiosity. Third, autonomy is not our only value. It is not necessarily always our highest or most inviolable value. Welfare is an important value too, and if life is so fucking great, maybe its greatness overrides the value of autonomy. This seems rather dubious to me, but maybe it would seem more persuasive to me if I thought that life was great. Fourth, we have a very strong biological and psychological interest in procreating. It is not something normally undertaken just to satisfy curiosity. The fact that refraining from procreation would be a great cost to many people is an important difference between procreation and the Peep experiment.

b) *Children: A (Liberal's) Nightmare:* Even though we can rebut Shiffrin's argument, a lingering liberal worry regarding children and autonomy remains. Liberals don't talk very much about children; as Herzog observes, liberals "would prefer we sprang full blown into the world, free agents from the start."[40] It is hard to know how to treat a person who is incompetent, but is also supposed to be nurtured and guided toward competence and autonomy, and grows continually and incrementally more capable of autonomy. We may try not to foreclose too many future exercises of autonomy, we may nurture rather than squelch our children's autonomy, but we still must face the fact that we make what may be the most important and riskiest decision of their lives entirely without their input. That degree of paternalism is uncomfortable, even if we have no way to consult the future person and even if life

40. Don Herzog, *Happy Slaves*, University of Chicago Press, 1989, 240.

is usually a pretty good experience and of reasonably high quality. When we add this worry to our worry that life is actually, or can be, possibly, not all that good (or even bad), it is not a worry easily resolved. It lingers.

IV   SUICIDE: GET OUT OF JAIL (AKA LIFE) FREE?

If suicide is painless, it may serve as a balm, of sorts, for our lingering procreative worries. Maybe children, or adults, who find that life is not worthwhile, can just kill themselves, thereby undoing our procreative errors. Suicide can give those upon whom life was thrust a way out. But, as many have noted, suicide is difficult and not just because one tends to get used to living.[41] It is scary because it forces a voluntary and foreseen confrontation with death, something we may be biologically programmed to avoid; it requires skill and knowledge, in the absence of which the attempter may be rendered worse off; and it usually causes great suffering to others. In fact, concern for the feelings of others may cause many who would otherwise commit suicide to continue to endure life. In this way, the loving relationships that are usually thought to enhance life may be the seal of doom, the kiss of life, so to speak: you may want to die, all things considered, but decide not to kill yourself because you don't want to make your loved ones suffer.[42] Yet parents cannot

---

41. See Benatar, *Better Never to Have Been*, 211–220 and Weinberg, "Is Having Children Always Wrong?"
42. The fact that one has loved ones does not entail that one's life is thereby made good or tolerable (for the opposite view, see Smilanksy, "Life Is Good"). In fact, the relationships with said loved ones might be entirely unsatisfying. You may not even like these people, yet you love them nonetheless and are too kind to put them through the misery and guilt of your suicide.

help by trying to make it easier for their children to commit suicide (should their children so choose) by being less loving toward them since then the parents can wind up being a contributing cause of their child's suicidal wishes. As a parent, you can't really occupy a neutral position regarding your child's possible suicide—a neutral position will likely serve as a positive reason to commit suicide (your own parents don't even care either way!). It looks like parents have no better choice but to play the role they generally play, that is, to act as reasons not to commit suicide, but those reasons are not always happy reasons or reasons that one is happy to have. Finally, the fact that so many people think that there is a life after death makes suicide less available as a procreative worry balm because many people believe that suicide will not result in the cessation of their experiences or existence. Even worse, some believe that committing suicide will commit them to eternal hell—the opposite of an escape from a life of suffering. Raising one's child to be an atheist is no guarantee that she won't grow to believe in an afterlife. There is no get-out-of-life-free card.[43]

V CONCLUSION

I have argued against the claim that life is an objectively bad experience and of low quality and that, therefore, procreation is almost

---

43. Even those who would prefer to have never been may not want to die either: "A man who wishes that he had not been born is mourning the dead. How can such a man mourn? He should covet the release! But he has been captured by the world. He didn't want to come and he doesn't want to go. And so he mourns." (Leon Wieseltier, *Kaddish*, Vintage Books/Random House, 1998, 223). For a particularly persuasive account of how one may prefer to never have been born even if one judges one's life worth living, see Saul Smilansky, "Preferring Not to Have Been Born," in *10 Moral Paradoxes*, Wiley-Blackwell, 2007.

always wrong. There is no accessible "objective" value of life experience for people, and the overwhelming majority of people value life in general and their own life in particular. I have also argued against the claim that procreation is almost always wrong because it violates the consent rights of future people. Procreation creates children, and children do not have consent rights. Thus, the two central lines of argument toward the conclusion that procreation is almost always wrong have serious flaws. We therefore cannot conclude that having children is almost always wrong.

Nevertheless, we are left with lingering worries. Maybe life is bad, or is bad enough, or risky enough, or uncertain enough, or scary enough, or unknown enough to make procreation almost always wrong. Maybe the person who does not appreciate life, particularly her own, will be your child. Maybe making the most important and far-reaching decision on behalf of another person is something we should not do, if we can help it, even if it doesn't violate anyone's consent rights. That is as far as I can progress on this question, and it is perhaps fitting to stop at this point. There are no strong and solid arguments against all procreativity, but there are lingering worries about whether it is almost always wrong anyway. That seems to indicate that if we do not have a strong interest in procreating, then we ought not to do so. It is the more morally conservative course of action.

Chapter 5

The Principles of Procreative Permissibility

Since it seems that procreation is not clearly almost always wrong and not clearly almost always right, we should try to figure out when procreation is permissible and when it isn't. There are many ways to go about doing this. My way is to take a broadly Kantian/ Rawlsian approach to determining principles of procreative permissibility. I will explain why I think that this way is especially suited to questions of procreative permissibility. I won't explain why I don't take alternate routes, such as consequentialism or virtue ethics (that's a whole other book). Instead, I will offer my approach and explain why I think it is theoretically appropriate and practically action-guiding. Although I argue for the principles of procreative permissibility on a contractualist basis, I believe that the principles can stand on their own, without contractualist support. They have intuitive appeal and are persuasive on the basis of simple fairness considerations, as I will argue. However, my view is that the contractualist method I use here makes the fairness and reasonableness of the principles more clear and provides an independent argument for their adoption. I therefore offer both the contractualist and the direct route to the principles of procreative permissibility.

I   WHY CONTRACTUALISM?

Contractualism views morality as a mutually respectful way of interacting with other people who are worthy of respect as ends in themselves. It presumes acknowledgment of the intrinsic moral worth of other people and the motivation to treat them with appropriate respect. Two key factors make contractualism a Kantian type of moral theory: the fact that it is based on the acknowledgment of persons as worthy of respect as ends in themselves and the fact that it requires and expects us to be motivated to treat people respectfully.[1]

(i) The Importance of Appropriate Motivation   Just as Kantian contractualism emphasizes the importance of being properly motivated, we have determined that proper procreative motivation is crucial to its permissibility. Proper procreative motivation is important because it helps to ensure that we are procreating in ways that are not disrespectful to children or inconsistent with our broadly liberal values of autonomy, respect, and equality (see Chapter 1). For example, procreating because one wants to engage in the parent-child relationship as a nurturing parent would be an acceptable procreative motive, but procreating to impress the neighbors would be a problematic procreative motive, regardless of outcome, because it does not

---

1. See Tim Scanlon, *What We Owe to Each Other*, Harvard University Press, 2000 and Stephen Darwall, *The Second-Person Standpoint*, Harvard University Press, 2009. See also John Rawls, *A Theory of Justice*, Harvard University Press, 1971. Rawlsian contractualism has a more complex motivational structure because it is multilayered. One embarks on Rawlsian contractualism motivated by a sense of justice and then, within the structure of the original position that Rawls uses as a thought experiment intended to arrive at principles of justice, one is instructed to select principles on a self-interested basis. This may lead some to think of Rawlsian motivation as self-interest, but that is a result of mistaking the thought experiment invoked as methodology for the theory for the overarching theory.

treat the future child as a person deserving of respect and value in her own right.

Perhaps even more importantly, being properly motivated to procreate is what gives us permission to procreate at all, considering how risky and unpredictable procreation is (for those procreated). Thus, in order to differentiate procreation from our Peeps creation experiment considered in Chapter 4, our procreative motivation can't be something like mere curiosity. It has to be more respectable and respectful, consistent with treating others as ends in themselves. Kantian contractualism stresses the primacy of appropriate and respectful motivation.

(ii) Adjudicating the Conflict of Interests Inherent to the Ethics of Risk Imposition As I have argued throughout this book, procreation is a case of risk imposition. Risk imposers have an interest in doing the act that imposes a risk; those they place at risk have an interest in avoiding any harms resulting from the imposition of the risk. In the procreative case, parents have an interest in procreating, which imposes various risks on their children. To assess when the risk is permissible to impose, we consider the cost to the parents of restricting their risk-imposing activity and the costs children may bear if parental procreative risk imposition ripens into a harm. We are thus engaged in adjudicating a distributive conflict of interests.

Although parents and children have many interests in common, in fundamental ways, procreation involves a conflict of parent/child interests. Prospective parents have an interest in procreating; future people have an interest in optimal birth conditions. The procreative conflict consists in the conflict of interests between existing people with an interest in procreating and future people with an interest in optimal birth conditions.

When people procreate under conditions that risk a less than optimal life for their future children (which turns out to be every case of procreativity), there's a conflict of interests between prospective parents and future children. Children have an interest in being born in optimal health, to parents who are appropriately motivated and optimally equipped to care for them. This set of interests conflicts with the interests in procreating held by parents whose children may not be born in optimal health and by parents who may not be appropriately motivated or optimally equipped to care for them. Prospective parents may have an interest in procreating when they are old, mentally ill, adolescent, impoverished, share defective genes, or are subject to political persecution. These circumstances will likely have a negative impact on their future child's life. Does that mean that they ought not procreate? It's a complicated *conflict* question because if the parents don't bear the procreative burden in these cases (by accepting restrictions to their procreativity), their children will (by having diseases, teenage parents, living in poverty, being persecuted, etc.).

It can feel disorienting to think of parents and children as having conflicting interests because we may be used to thinking of parents and children as natural allies, with many interests in common. Maybe, but procreative interests are not necessarily among them. Parents and children have many mutual interests once a child is born, but there are fewer points of mutuality before a child exists, when prospective parents may want to create children but their future children have no interest in being created and have an interest in optimal birth conditions should they be created. We need guidelines to help us adjudicate the procreative conflict justly and to fairly promote and protect prospective parental interests and the interests of future people.

Contractualism is designed to handle conflicts of interests, as it is fundamentally an account of how to interact with—how to make deals (contracts) with—others who are just as entitled to respect and autonomy as we are. How to balance what we want to pursue and how we wish to be treated with the rights and claims of others is a guiding point of all contractualist theories. The contractualist theory most directly aimed at adjudicating conflicts of interests is Rawlsian contractualism. That speaks in favor of it as a model for formulating our principles of procreative permissibility.

(iii) The Nature of Procreative Rights Violations Since Kantian/Rawlsian contractualism is a deontological theory, the wrong to children born to parents who have violated principles of procreative permissibility is that their parents failed to abide by just procreative principles. Rawlsian contractualism is a Kantian deontological theory that is principle rather than outcome based. Therefore, if, for example, the principle of procreative permissibility bars carriers of Huntington's disease from procreating, then the complaint that the person suffering from Huntington's would have is that her parents did not abide by just procreative principles. It is a rights-based claim. Once we set a procreative standard of care, any procreative act that does not conform to that standard violates the standard and violates the rights of people to have been procreated in accordance with that standard. One advantage of a principle-based standard of care is that we easily avoid non-identity kinds of challenges to procreative negligence, such as, "Yes, you have Huntington's disease, but your life is still worth living, so you have no procreative complaint." As argued in Chapter 3, people can have objections to having their rights violated even if those rights violations do not have a negative impact on their overall welfare status.

The objection is to the violation of the right and not to the negative impact on overall welfare status. (See Woodward's example of an African American who is denied an air ticket because of his race and the plane then crashes—the violation of his rights does not have a negative impact on his overall welfare status, but he still has grounds for a rights-based complaint.)[2] On my Rawlsian view, the complaint is a complaint about a rights violation regardless of the act's impact on the victim's overall welfare status.

II   WHY RAWLSIAN CONTRACTUALISM?

(i) Adjudicating Conflicts of Interests Unlike more recent Kantian contractualist theories, Rawlsian theory is focused more narrowly on adjudicating distributive conflicts of interests and formulating principles of distributive justice that will help construct the basic structure of a just society.[3] We can think of the procreative conflict as a distributive dilemma: How can we fairly distribute procreative benefits and burdens between prospective parents and future children? The Rawlsian way to answer that question is to ask yourself, "If I didn't know which person I would turn out to be, which rules would I choose to govern my society?" Rawls calls his metaphorical blinders, which we don in order to carry out this thought experiment, "the veil of ignorance."[4] The Rawlsian

---

2. James Woodward, "The Non-identity Problem," *Ethics* 1986 96: 804–83.

3. See Rivka Weinberg, "Procreative Justice: A Contractualist Account," *Public Affairs Quarterly* 2002 16: 405–425. Rawls addresses socioeconomic distributive conflicts of interests and seeks just principles to govern our socioeconomic and political institutions. Here, I seek morally just and respectful principles to (voluntarily) govern individual procreativity. But this difference does not seem to pose particular difficulties in applying a broadly Rawlsian framework, as we will see.

4. See Rawls, *A Theory of Justice*, 19.

thought experiment is intended to provide us with an especially compelling sort of impartiality. It begins with our thoughtful attempt to remove our natural bias toward ourselves and people like us by asking us to imagine that we don't know what sort of person we will turn out to be and then, from this veiled perspective, choose principles that our society will abide by. (Rawls intends for the principles to be part of the society's legal system and sociopolitical structure. I intend our principles here to be moral principles that moral individuals will, one hopes, choose to abide by.) The principles that we arrive at in this way, from what Rawls metaphorically calls "the original position,"[5] are compelling to us because their fairness is intuitive. We pick the principles ourselves, in a way that mitigates our bias toward ourselves and people like us. And it is obvious to us that this bias toward ourselves and people like us is a bias and not a legitimate partiality because we can see how imagining ourselves to be in a different societal role may change which rules we would pick. Thus, the Rawlsian thought experiment works to convince us of its fairness while we are in the process of engaging in it, and enables us to move closer to principled conflict resolution.

(ii) Defending the Veil Many object to the Rawlsian method of imagining that one could be anyone, in order to select just distributive principles, because we can't know what it's like to walk in someone else's shoes and also because we can't make choices without an identity from which to choose. (If I don't know who I am, how do I know what I want?)[6] Of course it's true that we cannot really *know* what it's like to be another

5. Rawls, *A Theory of Justice*, 12.
6. See Thomas Nagel, "Rawls on Justice," *Philosophical Review* 1973 82: 220–234.

person, and we certainly don't know what it is like to "be" no one. We are stuck, to some degree, in our own heads and in our own selves. The question is, to what degree, and how much does this matter to the Rawlsian thought experiment? If we were completely incapable of imagining things from another person's point of view, we would have a hard time with most moral reasoning and moral behavior. Moral reasoning generally seems to involve empathy and moral imagination. That's why it is common to teach children about basic morality by asking them, "How would you feel if someone grabbed your toy?" Imagining ourselves in another's shoes is probably not quite the same thing as actually finding ourselves there, but it is still an important method of understanding the viewpoint of others. Empathy and moral imagination are the tools we have for trying to understand different perspectives. Why not use them? It seems reasonable to try to do the best we can with the tools we have. It is not hopeless—if we were hopeless at seeing a situation from another person's point of view it is doubtful that we would ever develop much in the way of moral reasoning, moral principles, and moral behavior.[7] We also have the testimony of others, informing us of their perspective and giving

7. Individuals with autistic spectrum disorders are often referred to as lacking in empathy, yet they can engage in moral reasoning and behavior. This is puzzling only if we assume that autistic people have no empathy or moral imagination, but recent studies challenge these dubious claims. Recent studies indicate that individuals on the autistic spectrum have difficulties noticing and interpreting social and emotional cues from others, but they still do care for others and are capable of moral imagination and cognition, especially if educated. See Shari Hirvelä and Klaus Helkama, "Empathy, Values, Morality, and Asperger's Syndrome," *Scandinavian Journal of Psychology* 2011 52: 560–572; and Victoria McCeer, "Varieties of Moral Agency: Lessons from Autism (and Psychopathy)," in *Moral Psychology*, vol. 3: *The Neuroscience of Morality: Emotion, Brain Disorders, and Development*, Walter Sinnott-Armstrong, Ed., MIT Press, 2008, 227–258. See also Simon Baron-Cohen, *The Science of Evil: On Empathy and the Origins of Cruelty*, Basic Books, 2011; and Paul Bloom, "I'm O.K., You're a Psychopath," *New York Times*, June 17, 2011.

us some insight into what it is like to be like them. When we reason from behind the Rawlsian veil, our moral imagination is informed by the understanding gained by having listened to and read about the experiences of others with different talents, abilities, challenges, frustrations, interests, and desires. The veil does not blind us completely (to our interests or to the interests of others), of course; it just helps make our own particular interests much more hazy and the interests of others more clear, which helps us consider the interests of other people who have equal moral standing in a more equal way. It is a valuable theoretical device suited to our purposes.

III   OBJECTIONS TO THE RAWLSIAN CONTRACTUALIST METHOD FOR FORMULATING PRINCIPLES OF PROCREATIVE PERMISSIBILITY

(i) It's Impossible!—or Biased   In order to reason more fairly about procreative permissibility, the Rawlsian thought experiment directs us to imagine that we will be governed by the procreative principles we choose. Some argue that this thought experiment requires us to consider the possibility of our own nonexistence because if we assume that we will definitely exist, no matter which procreative principles we choose, we seem to have lost the fairness advantage gained by reasoning from a Rawlsian original position of ignorance about ourselves. If we know that we will definitely exist, we have nothing to lose by accepting very stringent procreative principles permitting procreation only under circumstances of extreme advantage and low risk to future people. (We won't exclude ourselves from existence and we will improve the nature of our existence, or at least of our birth

circumstances.) However, it is argued, we cannot really imagine that it might be true, in the actual history of the actual world, that we never exist.[8]

a) *Reply:* It's true that we cannot vividly imagine our own non-existence because there's no there there to think about. We can imagine a world that doesn't include us—that's a picture we can conjure up—but of course we can't imagine the state or event of our own nonexistence because that is no state at all and no event that befalls us. That picture is blank. But we can bypass this confusing thought process and simply accept, for the sake of argument, that in the procreative Rawlsian thought experiment we assume that we will exist. Does this render our reasoning biased or inappropriately partial? Will we indeed then have no reason not to adopt unreasonably stringent principles of procreative permissibility, given that we know that we will exist in any case?

I think not. The existent perspective is the appropriate one because, as argued in Chapter 3, only those who did, do, or will exist merit moral consideration. We don't have to save any birthday cake for our imaginary friends. Assuming our own existence is not a bias. We shouldn't consider the hypothetical interests of merely possible people. Merely hypothetical entities don't exist and don't matter. The procreative conflict of interests is about the procreative benefits and burdens born by real people. It's about the conflict between prospective parental interests in procreative freedom and future children's interests in optimal birth conditions. It is not an existence lottery or contest. Everyone gets to exist. When we engage in the Rawlsian procreative thought

8. See Derek Parfit, *Reasons and Persons*, Oxford University Press, 1984, 392–393.

experiment, we assume that we will exist but will have to abide by the procreative principles that we choose when it comes time for us to exercise our procreative capacities, and this will urge us away from unduly or unreasonably stringent principles of procreative permissibility.

When Parfit considers applying a Rawlsian method to procreative moral matters, he rejects the method as prejudicial:

> This [Rawlsian procreative] reasoning assumes that, whatever principle is followed, we shall certainly exist. This assumption violates the principle of impartiality. The principle we choose affects how many people exist. If we assume that we shall certainly exist whatever principle we choose, this is like assuming, when choosing a principle that would disadvantage women, that we shall certainly be men.[9]

But analysis of Parfit's analogy demonstrates his error. There are conflicts of interests and distributive justice tensions between men and women, and, therefore, assuming a male perspective may render any principles arrived at on the basis of that assumption unfairly partial. Existence, however, is not a distributable benefit: everyone has it and no one can lack it. There is no injustice in nonexistence because there are no (real) subjects for such an (hypothetical) injustice. Neither people in general nor individuals in particular will be disadvantaged by the assumption of an existent perspective. In contrast, women may be disadvantaged by the assumption of a male perspective. There are no conflicts of interests and no distributive justice tensions between hypothetically possible people that will turn out to exist

9. Parfit, *Reasons and Persons*, 392.

in the future (i.e., future people) and hypothetically possible people that will turn out not to exist in the future (i.e., merely possible people). So it is no prejudice to assume existence when considering principles of procreative permissibility. The procreative conflict is not about who is awarded the grand prize of existence. It is about whether people should have more procreative liberty or more optimal birth conditions when these sets of interests conflict.

Thus, although it may well be impossible to imagine the actual state of your own nonexistence, impartial consideration of the conflict of interests between prospective parents and future children does not require this kind of thinking because existence itself is not one of the interests involved in the procreative conflict. Existence itself is not being distributed. It is not a distributable benefit. (Everyone has it and no one can lack it.)

(ii) It Is Counterintuitive Some also argue that the assumption of existence will force us into counterintuitive choices. For example, Parfit argues that if we try to be Rawlsian contractualists about procreation and we assume that we will exist, then we are forced to choose an overpopulated hell (Hell I) that will last for forty-nine days and twenty-three hours over a less populated hell (Hell II), containing just a few people, but lasting fifty days. Since we will exist in either case, suffering for an hour less is what we would want even though, intuitively, Hell II is the obvious choice since it entails far less suffering overall. Yet, if we are choosing principles that will govern our own lives and we know that we will exist, it would make prudential sense for us to choose Hell I.[10]

10. Parfit, *Reasons and Persons*, 393.

a) *Reply:* Contractualism is an approach to the selection of moral principles; it is not an outcome-based theory, and it does not choose outcomes per se. A Rawlsian contractualist has very little to say about Hells I and II without knowing how and why these outcomes come to pass. One difference between a principle-based theory and an outcome-based theory is that outcome-based theories look to the result of an act to determine its permissibility, while principle-based theories look to the principle that an act accords with to determine its permissibility. Thus, according to Rawlsian contractualism, without knowing which principles result in Hell I or II, we have nothing to say about these cases.

Moreover, when we pick procreative principles we will try to respect and promote the interests of those affected by them. If a principle of procreative permissibility is likely to result in any sort of hell, that principle will presumably be rejected. If we are given a choice of procreative principles, one of which results in Hell I and the other of which results in Hell II, we will reject both as principles of procreative permissibility. It seems like any principle that results in hell for those living in accordance with it is a principle we would like to avoid. If hell is an inevitable result of procreativity, then the Rawlsian contractualist seeking principles of procreative permissibility would not choose Hell I over Hell II or Hell II over Hell I. Instead, she will choose a principle that bans procreation under hellacious conditions. That is the choice consistent with selecting principles that will govern oneself, whomever one turns out to be.[11]

11. There may be cases when procreation under hellacious conditions is permitted. This will depend, in part, on the cost to prospective parents of refraining from procreating. It is hard to imagine how this might work, though, because even if not procreating will result in a worse hell for the prospective parents than their children, hell is hell, and it is hard to see how one would choose a procreative principle that will allow procreation into hell just to make the hell that already existent people are in a slightly less hellacious hell.

IV   HOW RAWLSIAN CONTRACTUALISM?

I will now explain how we go about choosing principles of procreative permissibility that will govern ourselves, whomever we turn out to be.

(i) Parents or Children? We could try to choose principles that will govern us whether we turn out to be prospective parents or future children. This may seem simplest since these are the parties with conflicting procreative interests. But most future children will also grow into prospective parents, making it seem like we have one set of interests to consider rather than a conflicting set. And the one set we seem to have will skew our thinking toward parental interests because most children will become prospective parents, but prospective parents will not become children.[12] It might be more clear to just think of ourselves as being born, as children, under the principles we select and being governed, as prospective parents, by these same principles. This way of thinking about which principles of procreative permissibility we would want to govern us if we didn't know who we would be is straightforward: the principles we pick govern ourselves over the course of the various stages of our lives. They govern our birth and our procreativity. The conflict of interests that our principles will adjudicate, then, will be an *intrapersonal* rather than an *interpersonal* conflict: it will be the conflict between interests we have at different stages of life. As children, we have an interest in being born under favorable conditions, and, as prospective parents, we

12. If there's a conflict of interests between sets x and y, and the members of set x will usually become members of set y, then we seem to have reason to favor set y, and we also seem to have reason to think that there is no real conflict of interests here at all.

have an interest in being permitted to procreate under a very wide range of conditions, or simply whenever we feel like it. Since children, in the normal course, grow into prospective parents, the most accurate way to model the interpersonal procreative conflict may be to structure the hypothetical deliberation *intrapersonally*.[13]

Of course, we can't actually go back in time and recreate our birth conditions. This is a *hypothetical* thought experiment, intended to help us think clearly and with as little bias as possible. And so we *imagine* selecting principles of procreative permissibility that our parents will have abided by and that we, in turn, will be bound by as prospective parents. In a more typical contractualist scenario, we imagine an interpersonal conflict because we want to make sure that each party to the conflict is fully represented in our deliberations. For example, in creating an economic distribution principle, we might imagine that we could turn out to be a trapeze artist in a traveling circus or a stay-at-home mother, since we are unlikely to be both and each may have different economic interests. But in the procreative case, since we will each usually occupy both positions to the conflict, an intrapersonal conception of the conflict will not bias our decision-making. To the contrary, it may make our thought experiment easier to engage in since we need not imagine parts of a life in isolation. Instead, we imagine the natural course of a life, which begins in infancy, proceeds through adulthood, and ends in old age and death. We will try to select principles of procreative permissibility that take our interests during these various stages of life into appropriate account.

13. Just as in Rawls's thought experiment the deliberations can be thought of as being conducted by a sole deliberator, so too with the procreative thought experiment: we may think of the (intrapersonal) deliberations as conducted by a sole deliberator.

It may seem circular or question begging to assume that we will exist when we are selecting principles that will partly determine who will exist. But remember that we are not selecting *who* will exist at all. Instead, we are selecting *principles* of procreative permissibility (to be followed by prospective parents), and we assume that we will exist because the principles are supposed to apply to existent people. It's true that if the principles of procreative permissibility are followed, a different set of people will live than if they are not followed or if alternate principles are followed. This is true of almost every decision we make and every act we do (see Chapter 3), but it is of no moral significance here and of no metaphysical dishonesty to pay this fact no attention. We are engaging in a thought experiment designed to help us determine fair and unbiased *principles* of procreative permissibility. We appropriately imagine that we will exist—that is necessary if we are to merit moral consideration, and it is also what gives us a stake in the principles.

To clarify, our task is to compare how people who will exist under principle *x* fare as compared with how people who will exist under principle *y* fare and, imagining ourselves as a future person who will be born into and procreate under principle *x* or *y*, decide which principle we would choose: if we choose a principle that bans adolescent procreation, we will not be born to adolescents and we will not be permitted to procreate as an adolescent. Similarly, if we choose a principle that bans procreation with a 50% or greater chance of resulting in a child with Down syndrome, then we decrease our own chances of being born with Down syndrome to no more than 49%, and we restrict ourselves from procreating if our doing so has a 50% or greater chance of resulting in a child with Down syndrome. In this way, in our thought experiment, we select principles and imagine living in accordance with them. We compare life under various principles assuming that we will be *a* person but we don't know *which* person. Will we be the child born under high risk of Down syndrome and, therefore, quite possibly living with Down syndrome or the prospective parent who wants to procreate under a high risk of giving birth to a child with it? Our task is to imaginatively project what life would be like for us under various principles of procreative permissibility, not to predict or determine future population.[14]

(ii) The Veil When we ask ourselves which procreative principles we would choose if we did not know which person we would be, we need some general information in order to answer the question sensibly. For example, we need to know the statistics regarding birth conditions that increase with the age of the mother or father, such as Down syndrome, autism, and schizophrenia. We need to know about the effects of being a single parent or being the child of a single parent, and so on. We want to make an unbiased choice, not an ignorant one. Therefore, we will only try to blind ourselves (hypothetically) to biasing information, which, in this is case, is only personal identity information. We want to "see" the information about the probability of various procreative outcomes under various conditions. This knowledge is important for a few reasons. First, the impact of

---

14. Say we are living with a condition like cystic fibrosis and we choose a procreative principle that will require prospective parents to test for the genes that cause this condition and refrain from procreating if their future child could suffer from it. If we adopt that principle, then we don't exist? No. Of course we exist—we are conducting the experiment! What we are doing is choosing principles of procreative permissibility in an unbiased way, and it turns out that we choose a principle that tells us that our parents may well have done the wrong thing by creating us. Again, the important thing to remember is that we are choosing principles of procreative permissibility. We are selecting principles of procreative permissibility—we are not in the business of predicting or determining future population.

risking various birth outcomes varies with the kind of risk and the probability of the risk ripening into a harm; second, sometimes the incidence of a feature determines its impact (if most people over forty needed wheelchairs to get around, being wheelchair bound would be much easier because we would structure our societies to accommodate this widespread feature); and, finally, knowledge of procreative probabilities is important to help us choose realistic, persuasive principles that are neither too reckless nor too cautious.[15]

Thus, we will take societal and species information into account. We veil knowledge of which person we will turn out to be so we don't know which society we will be born into, but we will want to know the nature and degree of variation of societal norms, customs, and attitudes. This will help us select principles that are applicable across cultures and sensitive to cultural differences (e.g., dyslexia is not as disadvantageous in an agrarian society as it is in a literate, industrialized society). It will also help us focus on disadvantage in societies as they are and not as they might be if we put more effort into mitigating disabilities, though we may still choose principles that will work better if such mitigation efforts are undertaken and even consider whether our principles will encourage such mitigation. On the flip side, we will have to consider that restricting procreation under certain circumstances

15. Rawls veils knowledge of probabilities in his original position, assigning his deliberators an equal chance of being anyone even though some identities are more likely than others. However, Rawls's veiling of probabilities has resulted in many charges of question begging, especially by consequentialists who argue that it is only this move that allows Rawls's deliberators to avoid choosing average utility as the principle of justice. See R. M. Hare, "Rawls's Theory of Justice," in *Reading Rawls*, Norman Daniels, Ed., Stanford University Press, 1989. (Many think that this principle would be chosen anyway from Rawls's original position, even if probabilities remain veiled. See Hare, "Rawls's Theory of Justice.") By not veiling probabilities here, I avoid similar question-begging charges.

may reduce the incidence of certain conditions and ultimately make those conditions more difficult to live with because they will become more rare and, hence, likely less attended to by society. We will also know what we can know about being human; for example, it is normal for humans to see, usually optimal for humans to have 20/20 vision, and disadvantageous for humans to be blind. This will help us understand the nature and extent of various abilities and conditions.

(iii) Procreative Goods So we sit, veiled, trying to figure out which principles of procreative permissibility to choose to govern our lives, assuming we don't know which person we will turn out to be. What, then, do we want from a principle? Why choose one over another? What is good for us?

We don't know who we will be, so we will have to make sure that what we are aiming at has very wide appeal. Presumably, it is good for everyone to lead a rich, rewarding, happy, moral, meaningful life. But which procreative goods increase our odds for attaining that sort of (desirable) life of human flourishing? Well, for starters, we will want to have our biological and psychological needs met: we will want to be well nourished, in good mental and physical health, well educated, socially connected, have self-respect, and not be oppressed. Procreative goods are basic human goods that seem foundational to further pursuit of what each person might, on their own and as they mature, determine to be a good life. Beyond these basic, foundational goods, it is optimal to be optimally nourished, in optimal health, optimally educated (i.e., in accordance with your abilities and interests), optimally socially connected (i.e., in accordance with your preferences and personality), have high self-respect and self-esteem, and be politically and personally free from oppressive forces. These goods seem to hold for all: given a choice, who would choose, ceteris paribus, to be hungry, sick, ignorant, self-hating, lonely, and oppressed? No one in her right mind. Although some may resist claiming that anything is good for everyone, the goods I have delineated are general enough to apply to everyone, unless one insists on a dogmatic and radical individualism, which seems strained to me given that people, for all of their variety, do have many biological and psychological features in common.[16]

Of the procreative goods listed here, the way procreative liberty is accounted for is, first, in terms of social connection. The parent-child relationship is a basic source of social connection on its own, and it also connects parents to other parents and to their society. Procreative liberty is an aspect of personal freedom and, as such, is also included in the good of not being oppressed. Self-respect is impacted by procreative liberty as well since having children is often a source of pride for people and, in some societies, not having children can cause a real or perceived loss of prestige that, in turn, may affect self-respect.

From behind our veil of ignorance, we won't want our conception of procreative goods to be more specific, because specific

16. For a far more detailed and thoroughgoing discussion of human goods, see Amartya Sen, *Commodities and Capabilities*, Oxford University Press, 1985; and Martha Nussbaum, "Human Capabilities, Female Human Beings," in Jonathan Glover and Martha Nussbaum, Eds., *Women, Culture, and Development*, Oxford University Press, 1995.

Compare this with the lack of objectivity we found in Chapter 4, when we attempted to evaluate the nature of human experience. We are all stuck inside human experience and have no authoritative position from which to issue a global, objective evaluation of it. In contrast, we can say with some degree of objectivity that some things are good for people, like having nutritional needs met. We can stand outside a starving person and make that kind of evaluative claim, from our position of nonstarvation.

goods apply to specific people and we don't know which specific person we will turn out to be. We don't know if we will want a baseball, a paintbrush, a donut, a church, or a library, but we do know that it would be nice to have a range of these kinds of choices, the freedom to choose how to express ourselves, and the self-respect to value ourselves and our choices. If this sounds somewhat individualistic, it is. Some might argue in favor of more communal values and goods, but if you don't know who you will be, sticking with an individualistic conception of the good is more prudent because it's more inclusive. Individualism does not preclude or foreclose communalism, so long as the communal affiliation is freely chosen or reflectively endorsed. If you think communes or kibbutzim or collective farms are more valuable or good than alternatives, go ahead and join one of these groups. An individualistic conception of the good used when deliberating in the original position will not stop you. It will only ensure your freedom to choose.[17] Since individualism allows you to join a commune but communalism usually doesn't let you out of one, individualism is the more inclusive choice. If you don't know who you will turn out to be, the more inclusive option is the prudent one.[18]

---

17. One might argue that, given the choice, people rarely choose the greater good of communalism. But if individuals tend not to make communal choices, then it is likely that communalism does not serve individuals very well. And we are all individuals, even though we are social beings.

18. Rawls assigns the deliberators in his original position a focus only on "primary goods" (*A Theory of Justice*, 95), i.e., goods necessary for any rational life plan. This makes sense for deliberators ignorant of which rational life plan they will choose (Rawls has other reasons for this conception of the good as well). But, in the procreative case, part of what is being distributed is the ability to have a wider set of primary goods be useful to one's range of life plans and also to have a greater choice set of rational life plans from which to choose. Therefore, primary goods are too narrow a conception of procreative goods for purposes of deliberating regarding principles of procreative permissibility.

(iv) Procreative Decision Principle While engaged in our procreative thought experiment, we don't know which person we will turn out to be, but we know that an abundance of procreative goods is good for us. It's good for us to have optimal health, nourishment, education, opportunities for social connection, and freedom. We will try to choose principles that maximize our chances of attaining high levels of important procreative goods. This differs from a straightforwardly utilitarian maximizing principle that would just tell us to seek the maximum level of good, period, in that we have defined procreative goods in ways that implicate rights, prioritize individual over collective good, and resist complete maximization because they are not entirely fungible. For example, the good of living free of oppression is very important and there will be times when it seems rational to risk some level of nourishment or shelter comforts for greater freedom of speech, association, or self-expression, but it's not like more freedom always makes up for less nourishment.

Another important example of a nonfungible and individualistic procreative good is the good of basic self-respect. Self-respect is not an all-or-nothing affair. One instance of "selling out" or being demeaned is unlikely to destroy your self-respect forever, but not being able to develop a healthy sense of self-respect in the first place may make you unable to ever attain a reasonable or threshold level of self-respect. Basic, threshold-level self-respect is a crucial good that is pervasive and worthy of special protection because it is the basis for valuing one's well-being.[19] If you don't value yourself, why would you value your own good? Because self-respect is fundamental to valuing oneself and one's good, it is prudent to pay special attention to protecting self-respect.

---

19. See Elizabeth Anderson, *Value in Ethics and Economics*, Harvard University Press, 1993, 59–60.

In my view, protecting the procreative good of basic self-respect requires that one's well-being won't be sacrificed solely for the sake of others or for the so-called "common good," such as being created as a source of organs for needy recipients. It is imprudent to risk being sacrificed because even though statistics dictate that if we sacrifice the few for the many, we are more likely to be benefited than burdened by the sacrifice (since we are more likely to be one of the many), living in a society that sanctions treating some as the mere means for the good of others puts self-respect at risk because it does not recognize people as selves at all. If we allow individual good to be sacrificed for the so-called "common good," then we are sanctioning the treatment of persons as expendable parts of a collective rather than as self-standing beings, deserving of respect in their own right. Being treated as a separate self, worthy of respect in one's own right, is important for basic self-respect because in order to have self-respect, one must have a robust sense of self to respect. You need to think of yourself as a "self" in order to have self-respect, as the term "*self*-respect" implies. And, in order to have a robust sense of self, one must generally be treated and considered as such. If you can be sacrificed for others, then you're not being treated as a separate self; instead, you are being treated as an expendable part of some other whole. A society that sanctions sacrifice treatment threatens threshold, basic-level self-respect because it undermines the conception of persons as separate selves, worthy of respect in their own right and for their own sake, that is, as "selves."[20]

20. This applies even to the possible attempt by a society to maximize the degree to which self-respect is secured, overall, because the collective nature of that attempt ends up treating individuals as mere means to the overall good of self-respect rather than as separate selves (one individual's self-respect could be sacrificed for the greater self-respect of a few others) entitled to self-respect in their own rights, as ends in themselves, and not as mere means to any other end, even the end of securing self-respect in a society.

We will want our principles of procreative permissibility to reflect the nature of procreative goods. That means that we will want to attain a variety of procreative goods (because they are not entirely fungible, a high level of one good will not necessarily make up for an extremely low level of another) and pay special attention to the special procreative good of basic self-respect. Our principles will have to reflect the rights and individualism implicated by our conception of procreative goods. They will also have to have some degree of rational flexibility since there is more than one rational approach to risk and since we don't have a completely ranked, fungible list of goods. It is not a subjective free-for-all, though. Some approaches to risk are irrational, and our principles should reflect that. For our purposes, I will use the term "irrational" to indicate that *everyone* has decisive reasons to avoid an act or decision.

V   THE PRINCIPLES OF PROCREATIVE PERMISSIBILITY

(i) Motivation Restriction Because we value self-respect, we will want to make sure that we are each treated as a separate person, worthy of respect in our own right, from the get-go. This means that:

> Procreation must be motivated by the desire and intention to raise, love, and nurture one's child once it is born.

Motivation is complex and behavior can be multiply motivated. All the Motivation Restriction requires is that the proper procreative motive—the parental motive, as discussed in Chapter 1, and delineated here—be present and prominent among one's procreative motivations. Procreation wholly otherwise motivated threatens our baseline, threshold level of self-respect because it is not respectful of each person as a separate person in her own right, entitled to respect and value for her own sake. Procreation primarily to generate help on the family farm, for example, threatens the future child's self-respect because it fails to consider her as a separate self, entitled to love, respect, and consideration in her own right. It will be hard for a child to develop basic self-respect if she is not treated as a self worthy of respect, and motivations generally affect outcomes. Empirical research supports these commonsense suppositions.[21]

The Motivation Restriction requires prospective parents to be motivated to treat their child as a separate person in her own right,

---

21. Narcissistic or exploitive parents are paradigm examples of parents who treat their children as extensions of themselves or as mere instruments for their own purposes. Their children have particular difficulty developing a sense of self and, therefore, healthy self-respect because they haven't been valued and treated as separate selves by their parents. See Sophie Lowenstein, "An Overview of the Concept of Narcissism," *Social Casework* 1997 58: 136–142; and Annie Reich, "Pathological Forms of Self-Esteem Regulation," *Psychoanalytic Study of the Child* 1960 15: 215–232. See also Elan Golomb, *Trapped in the Mirror: Adult Children of Narcissists in Their Struggle for Self*, William Morrow, 1992. There is not much research regarding the effects of procreative motivation and parent-child outcomes, but the little there is supports the view that motivation usually affects outcomes. The notion that parenthood itself creates or somehow brings out every person's innate proper parenting motivations is overly romantic and false. In most areas of human behavior, motivation affects outcome, and although motivation can change, it often doesn't. A 1999 University of Michigan study compared the relationship between intentional mothers and their children and unintentional mothers and their children. Unintended children were found to negatively significantly impact the relationship between the mother and the unintended child as well all of her other children (both intended and unintended). Mothers with unintended children were more likely than other mothers to slap or spank their children, and they were less likely to take their children on activities and trips outside the home, e.g., the park, movies, the zoo. Mothers with unintended children were also found to be less supportive of their adult children than other mothers, providing their young adult children with less help with childcare, moving, etc. or even simply talking. This study supports the pragmatic perspective: we want what we want and motivation affects outcomes. (See J. S. Barber, W. G. Axinn, and A. Thornton, "Unwanted Childbearing, Health, and Mother-Child Relationships," *Journal of Health and Social Behavior* 1999 40: 231–257.)

entitled to love and respect intrinsically, for herself, and not merely derivatively, through love or concern for themselves. If we don't know which person we will turn out to be, we will want to adopt this principle because it protects us from disregard for ourselves and our special good of self-respect. In turn, it demands that we only procreate when properly motivated ourselves. That is a worthwhile trade because basic self-respect, as argued, is fundamental and crucial. It is certainly not worth risking for the very dubious privilege of being permitted to procreate in ways inconsistent with respecting one's child for her own sake.

a) *Compelling in Its Own Right:* The Motivation Restriction makes sense on its own terms as well, regardless of contractualist considerations per se. We have no moral excuse to procreate disrespectfully. Just as we treat existing persons with respect, just as we want to be treated with respect, we should treat future persons with respect. It is not controversial to think this even though it may have some controversial implications when applied to contemporary savoir sibling cases, historical help-on-the-farm cases, or the like. I will take up these sorts of cases in more depth in Chapter 6.

(ii) Procreative Balance In our attempt to maximize our procreative goods and realize our procreative interests over the course of our lifetimes, it will be instructive to note where the tensions between our earlier and later procreative interests lie. It is easier to spot the points of tension working backward, from our interest in procreative liberty to our interest in being born with a very high level of procreative goods. For example, we may want to have the freedom to delay procreation until our early forties in order to give us time to establish ourselves in our careers. But, if our procreative principle permits that, then we have a significantly higher risk of

being born with significant health problems since the risk of many serious genetic problems rises significantly with parental age and our parents will have abided by a principle permitting delayed procreativity. This is the sort of balancing that our principle of Procreative Balance will guide.

The principle of Procreative Balance tells us to consider whether it is rational for us to risk being born with disadvantage x in exchange for the permission to procreate under condition y. This is consistent with our Rawlsian contractualist approach: we are trying to pick a principle that will maximize our procreative goods over the course of our lifetimes, and it makes prudential sense to do so by balancing our different procreative interests at different times of our lives. So, to continue the prior example, we might ask ourselves if being born with a 100% greater chance of having Down syndrome is worth the permission to delay procreation from thirty-six to thirty-nine years old,[22] taking into account both the increase in risk and the actual risk (if the risk doubles but remains miniscule, the fact that the risk doubles will not be as salient). We can formalize these kinds of considerations with the following principle:

> Procreation is permissible when the risk you impose as a procreator on your children would not be irrational for you to accept as a condition of your own birth (assuming that you will exist), in exchange for the permission to procreate under these risk conditions.

---

22. At maternal age thirty-six, the risk of carrying a fetus with Down syndrome is one in two hundred; at thirty-nine it is one in one hundred. See Ernest B. Hook, Philip K. Cross, and Dina M. Schreinemachers, "Chromosomal Abnormality Rates at Amniocentesis and Live-Born Infants," *Journal of the American Medical Association* 1983 249: 2034–2038.

Thus, in the example we are considering, if it would be not be irrational to accept twice the risk of Down syndrome, from one out of two hundred to one out of one hundred, as a condition of your own birth in exchange for the permission to delay procreation from thirty-six to thirty-nine to better establish your career, then that delay would be permitted by the principle of Procreative Balance. If the risk is irrational to accept, then that sort of procreative delay would not be permissible. Whether the risk is irrational to accept will depend on how likely a negative outcome is, how your procreative birth goods will be impacted by a negative outcome, and how your procreative liberty goods will be impacted by procreative restriction (i.e., being denied permission to delay procreation from thirty-six to thirty-nine for career enhancement). I will apply this principle to some key cases in Chapter 6.

The principle of Procreative Balance will direct us to assess the impact of various degrees of procreative restriction against the impact of various degrees of risk to our various procreative birth goods. Procreation can either be banned entirely or only biologically (leaving open the possibility of adopting children) and can be restricted as to timing and number of instances. We may also consider whether refraining from sexual intercourse might ever be required due to lack of available birth control. The higher cost to the prospective parent in that sort of case would be taken into appropriate consideration. Procreative birth goods can be reduced from a level that renders the child capable of a life of human flourishing to that of human subsistence, or human suffering and abjection. The possibility and availability of preimplantation genetic diagnosis (PGD) and selective implantation of embryos may be considered as well. PGD may mitigate otherwise problematic procreativity when used, for example, to select non-Tay-Sachs-afflicted embryos but might seem to problematize otherwise less problematic procreativity when used to select for deaf or male embryos. These factors give us a lot to consider, and we will take up these issues in Chapter 6.

Why not be more straightforward, one might wonder, and simply ask whether it would be irrational for you to accept for yourself the risk you are imposing on your future child, in order to have a child at this point? If your child runs a 50% risk of being deaf, you might ask yourself whether it would be irrational for you to risk a 50% chance of going deaf in order to have a child. That may sometimes be a helpful way to think through a procreative dilemma, but it is subject to distortion because being deaf from birth (due to your parents' choice or not) is a different experience from going deaf in adulthood (due to your own choice to assume that risk). The purpose of this principle is to help us balance our interests in procreative liberty as prospective parents against our interests in being born with a set of optimal procreative goods. The most realistic way to think about that is to consider our interest in procreating under given risk conditions in balance with our interest in being born with optimal procreative goods.

a) *Compelling in Its Own Right:* Like the Motivation Restriction, the principle of Procreative Balance is compelling on its own terms, regardless of contractualist considerations.

• *Fair:* It is a model of fairness in that it shows us how to distribute procreative risks in ways that respect people's changing interests over the natural course of a lifetime. As intended, it turns out to provide us with an especially compelling impartiality, taking relevant interests into appropriate account, and bringing the interests of (prospective) parents and (future) children into sharp relief. This will be demonstrated further in Chapter 6, as we apply the principle to procreative cases. By weighing parental and child interests against each other, we can appreciate their nature and importance and make a rational cost-benefit type of prudential choice (within the constraints of the Motivation Restriction).

• *Flexible:* The principle of Procreative Balance is flexible, demanding more of parents who can do better by their children because that demand will cost the parents less and demanding less of parents with lesser resources. The following set of examples illustrate this point:

The Students: Mary and Joseph are Americans in their second year of college. They are eager to become parents and, given their carefree, relaxed personalities, are prone to be inconsistent about birth control. They figure that if they have a baby, they will be delighted to care for it and it will be okay. They are also aware that if they delay procreation until they complete their college education, they are far more likely to actually finish college and that college graduates in the United States earn significantly more money than nongraduates.[23] It can make the difference between managing to remain middle class or not.

The Home Health Aides: Bob and Barbara are thirty-three-year-old home health aides who live and work in California. Their salaries are fairly low; their children will not be middle class, but their basic needs will likely be met. If they could only have children with a very high chance of being born into

---

23. College graduates earn 84% more than high school grads, according to a 2011 study. See Anthony P. Carnevale, Stephen J. Rose, and Ban Cheah, "The College Payoff: Education, Occupations, Lifetime Earnings," Georgetown University Center on Education and the Workforce.

circumstances conducive to a life of human flourishing, that is, having a high or optimal level of procreative goods, they probably would have to refrain from procreating altogether.

Procreative Balance would require the college students to delay procreation, given that the benefit of remaining undisciplined about birth control is small compared to the difference their delay will likely make to their child's chances of achieving a life of human flourishing (as opposed to subsistence or worse). It would be irrational to risk giving up the many ways in which being middle class in the United States enhances the procreative goods of health, education, freedom, and nourishment for the freedom to be sloppy about birth control for two years. But Procreative Balance would permit the home health aides to procreate in this case because it is not irrational to risk a life of lesser flourishing, and possibly subsistence-level living, for the freedom to procreate under circumstances where having no children at all is the only other choice. Not having children is a high cost and is higher still if fewer alternate routes to fulfillment and flourishing are available.

Of course, these are relatively easy cases. But I use them to illustrate the flexibility of Procreative Balance. Harder cases will be addressed in Chapter 6.

• **Pluralistic:** Procreative Balance is general in its conception of procreative goods, specifying broad categories of things that are good for everyone and goods that can be expressed in a variety of ways. For example, being well educated means different things in different times and places—it can mean knowing which berries are poisonous or understanding the themes in *Paradise Lost*—but it is always good for people to have ample opportunity to become educated in the knowledge of their time and culture. Procreative Balance is not unduly narrow or restrictive, allowing for varying conceptions of the good and varying approaches to risk, constrained by the boundaries of rationality. So long as the risk is not assessed as *irrational*, procreation is deemed permissible. This allows for the many rational approaches to risk; we are not forced to be highly risk averse or reckless. But we can't just do anything and call it rational. There are enough cases of clear irrationality, as we saw in The Students' case and as we will see in some of the cases discussed in Chapter 6, to make Procreative Balance a useful and action-guiding principle. Where different rational approaches to risk occur, we err on the side of liberty and permit procreation. This is consistent with our broadly liberal, Kantian contractualist framework which places high value on autonomy. So long as a risk would not be irrational to take, the risk is permitted by Procreative Balance. It is a moderate, pluralistic principle, which I take to be an advantage, both in terms of its theoretical plausibility and in terms of its practical value. As with most general rules, however, we can expect exceptions to Procreative Balance and some cases where the principle will seem inadequate.

b) *Dramatic Comebacks, Happy Endings, and Seizings of the Day:* We are trying to maximize our procreative goods throughout the course of our lifetimes (within the constraints of the Motivation Restriction). Procreative Balance directs us to do this by balancing our interests in procreative goods at different stages of our lives. As children, we want optimal procreative goods; as adults, we want procreative liberty. We try, within the limits of rationality, to keep these conflicting interests in balance. This implies that we give no greater weight to one time of life, in and of itself, than to another.[24] Without knowing whom we turn out to be and how long we live, this seems the prudent choice. But there are challenges to this way of thinking about rational prudence. I will now address these challenges. Spoiler alert: the challenges will be disputed and defeated.

• **Dramatic comebacks:** Many a moving biography begins with a terrible childhood, followed by a dramatic or even heroic overcoming or persevering. It's exciting. Some find it inspiring as well. One might wonder whether it would be rational to value significant childhood deprivation since if we can overcome it, our lives would be even better than they'd be if we had a humdrum, boring, suburban, happy childhood. It would certainly make for a better *story*. However, that doesn't mean that it would make for a better life. (Happiness does not make for an interesting read, yet most people enjoy experiencing it anyway.) Significant deprivation, especially in early childhood, usually has significant negative effects that are usually not overcome. One of the reasons why comeback tales are dramatic is that comebacks are unexpected. Great odds are usually not overcome. So it is not rationally prudent to undervalue one's early life procreative goods or to value childhood deprivation. The childhood stage of life has very significant effects on the rest of life's stages. Should we value it more highly, then, than later stages of life? Not in and of itself, since the only reason that childhood is particularly significant is because it usually has significant impact on later stages of life. Thus, childhood is no more important per

---

24. Although we give equal weight to all times of life, we do not average out the good by dividing the amount of good over the length of the lifetime and then favor the life with the greatest ratio because that could lead to the absurd preference of an extremely short but ecstatic life, e.g., a five-minute thrill, over a good eighty-year life.

se than other times of life, but we will want to pay attention to the effects of childhood on later stages of life so that we don't undervalue childhood procreative goods or interests and are realistic about the lifelong effects of childhood.

• *Happy endings:* Some argue that, like a feel-good movie, a good life needs a happy ending.[25] It's sad when lives end bitterly, and sometimes it seems sad enough to cast a pall on the entire life of the person. This can make it seem like the end of life is more important than other times of life. It's your last chance at a happy ending. But even if your life is, in a sense, a story you tell yourself, that does not mean that the elements that make a story good make for a good or desirable life. Good stories have lots of tension, drama, suspense, and dynamism. Good lives much less so. Furthermore, it seems to me that most lives don't end all that well. We usually don't go down in a blaze of glory. Instead, we tend to fizzle out in a painful progression of losses unless we get hit by a truck first. It is not easy to know what might reliably make life end well and not clear that doing so would be worth the cost. We could shoot ourselves in the head immediately following a high point, but that seems to irrationally overvalue the end. Thus, it seems rational to plan for old age and to do our best to mitigate its losses and difficulties, but it seems irrational to value old age more than any other stage of life merely because it is the last one. Given that many are not all that aware at life's end, it seems less prudent still to overvalue it due to its

---

25. David Velleman discusses the value of the narratives we tell ourselves about our lives and argues that the narratives are told retrospectively, looking back. It is a particular perspective from which a happy ending may be especially valuable, granting meaning and purpose to earlier struggle. But narrative retrospection is not the perspective of rational prudence. We plan our lives prospectively and from the forward-looking, planning perspective, we should take care not to overvalue or oversentimentalize life's end. See David Velleman, "Well-Being and Time," *Pacific Philosophical Quarterly* 1991 72: 48–71.

retrospective significance. Many of us will be incapable of retrospection or telling ourselves our life story, with its happy or sad ending, by the time we are at our (demented) life's end. As with life's beginning, we may include the retrospective significance of the end of life in our consideration of our well-being at the end of life, and that will lend the end of life a particular sort of significance, but it would not be rational to overvalue the nature and importance of a happy ending. And since the beginning and middle of life will, to a significant extent, inform and impact the end of our lives, the prudential rationality of valuing all times of life pretty much equally is further supported.

• *Seizing the day, discounting the future:* Some argue that it is rational to discount the future and to value the present more highly than other times of life. We seem to care most about something while experiencing it, they note. Pain is a good example of this: we mind pain most, care about it most, while suffering it.[26] It seems crazy not to. But this is only because minding something or caring about it is different from granting it prudential value. We can care about something in the emotional sense of caring without valuing it in the prudentially rational sense of considering it prudentially worthwhile. When the chocolate cake is tempting us, we desire it most while gazing at it longingly, enjoy it most—that is, care about it *emotionally*—while eating it, and regret it most—*prudentially*—after eating it. When in the dentist chair, we can emotionally care very much about our discomfort and grant it a lot of emotional value, but we don't grant it more prudential value just because it is happening to us *now*. If that were true, we'd get out of that chair. But we don't. We sit there and hold our mouths wide open, enduring the discomfort,

26. See Parfit, *Reasons and Persons*, 145–195 and 313–317.

because we don't grant the current discomfort greater prudential value just because it is in the present. We value all times of
life roughly equally, so we willingly endure a lesser discomfort
now to prevent a greater discomfort in the future. If it were really
rational to grant the present greater prudential value, we would
not necessarily conclude that a lesser current pain is preferable
to a greater later pain. But reasoning about present and future
trade-offs by deeming a lesser present pain worth the avoidance
of a greater future pain epitomizes prudential rationality, and it
does so precisely because it is prudentially irrational to be biased
toward the present.

The only sense in which it is prudentially rational to discount
the future is the extent to which you might die before the future
occurs. That's why I was immediately persuaded by my colleague Dion Scott-Kakures's reason for teaching his required five
classes a year by teaching two in the fall and three in the spring:
that way, if he dies in the fall, he will not have given the college
something for nothing. If you are going to die the next day, you
might as well leap out of the dentist chair and wolf down the
cake. An actuarial table will tell us the degree to which it is rational for us to discount the future by providing us with a statistical
analysis of when we are likely to die. But, actuaries aside, when
someone is dying and in pain, say, it is irrational to worry about
whether upping her narcotic dose will make it more likely she
will become addicted to the narcotic. Similarly, when people are
very old, it is irrational to worry too much about their diet. (Let
them eat cake.) Other than that, ceteris paribus, it is rational to
grant roughly equal value to all times of life, keeping in mind the
effects that some times have on others, the value of anticipation,
and the value of retrospection. No time has greater value per se
over another.

c) *Third-Party Considerations:* Notably, the principle of Procreative Balance only takes the interests of parents and their children into account. It does not attend to third-party considerations, for example, the state that needs youth to maintain society, culture, and productivity; the gravely ill sibling in desperate need of compatible bone marrow; people longing to be grandparents; members of dying cultures; and so on. These sorts of third-party considerations are a very complex matter that merit far more attention than I will give them here, mostly because I am exploring procreative ethics from the individual perspective of prospective parents and future children. I leave a full discussion of third-party concerns for another endeavor.

However, some third-party considerations are addressed or even settled by our procreative principles. Take the case of Down syndrome. If most people avoid having children with Down syndrome (via reduced risk pregnancy or by testing for and aborting Down-affected fetuses), then people living with the syndrome and those who care for them will suffer. They will suffer a loss of peers and society. They will also likely suffer from a loss of programs that address their needs and from reduced Down-related research since they will likely have fewer advocates. These are very serious difficulties to face. But I don't think it changes the permissibility of procreating with a high risk of Down syndrome in cases where such procreativity could be avoided at little cost to the prospective parents. Imagine a case of parents considering having a fifth child when they are both in their midforties. Their chances of having a child with Down syndrome are more than 5%.[27] Down

---

27. See Hook, Cross, and Schreinemachers, "Chromosomal Abnormality Rates." The mother's age in this case results in a 5% chance of having a child with Down syndrome. The father's age increases it significantly, though it is not yet known by exactly how much (see H. Fisch, G. Hyun, et al., "The Influence of Paternal Age on Down syndrome," *Journal of Urology* 2003 169: 2275–2278).

syndrome makes flourishing very challenging due to the significant cognitive and physical health limitations posed by the condition.[28] It's hard to see how it would not be irrational to run a significant risk of being born with Down syndrome in exchange for the freedom to permissibly create one's fifth child. Having four rather than five children has a minimal impact on a person's ability to lead a life of human flourishing (it restricts freedom, but does not seem to negatively impact other procreative goods). Could the fact that the Down community needs members make procreativity permissible in this case? Probably not. That would be tantamount to sacrificing a person for the sake of society, treating persons as mere members of a greater whole and not as selves, valuable in their own right and for their own sake. To create a person with a disability for the sake of existing people with that disability is similar to taking a healthy infant and giving her Down "pills" at birth (if that were possible) or like taking a hearing newborn and deliberately destroying her hearing in order to maintain the viability of the deaf community.[29] While living without peers or watching your culture die out around you is tragic, this tragedy does not justify drafting people to be your peers or to participate in your culture. It is, of course, possible that I have overlooked

28. Down syndrome causes mental retardation (IQ averages from 40 to 77). Other conditions associated with Down syndrome include congenital heart defects (common), gastrointestinal abnormalities (12%), risk of leukemia (10%–30% higher than the general population but still less than 1%), congenital cataracts (common), glaucoma (common), significant hearing loss, increasing with age (75%), thyroid dysfunction (40%), infertility (virtually all males, 70%–85% of females), and accelerated aging (see Janet Stewart, "Down Syndrome/Trisomy 21," *Genetic Drift: Management of Common Genetic Disorders*, 1998 16, web). Nearly all people with Down syndrome have Alzheimer's pathology by age forty (See "Down Syndrome and Alzheimer's Disease," Alzheimer's Association, *Alz.org*, web). Treatment has improved quality of life outcomes but has not reduced the incidence of the above-noted aspects of the syndrome.

29. The non-identity fact that these children would not exist without Down syndrome is, as argued in Chapter 3, of no moral relevance.

some important considerations here, and it is almost certain that, in some cases, third-party interests make a moral difference, but I do not address those issues here.

VI COMPARING PRINCIPLES

More Compelling Than Competing Principles The principles of procreative permissibility for which I have argued makes sense on their own terms and are supported by Kantian and Rawlsian contractualist theory. They also are more fair, more practical, and more reasonable than the alternatives that have been proposed, as I will now argue.

(i) Birthright Principles Some philosophers have argued that children have the right to be born into circumstances of "minimal decency." They argue that this birthright is violated when children are created by parents who can foresee that their children are unlikely to born into minimally decent conditions.[30]

The problem with birthright principles is that they are problematically vague, giving us little guidance regarding what counts as minimal decency. They are also inflexible and, in that sense, unfair in that they demand the same level of procreative goods for children regardless of the parents' ability to secure it. If parents can secure a much higher level of procreative goods for their children at little or no cost to themselves, why not demand more?

---

30. See Joel Feinberg, "Wrongful Life and the Counterfactual Element in Harming," *Social Philosophy and Policy* 1986 4: 145–179; and Bonnie Steinbock, "The Logical Case for Wrongful Life," *Hastings Center Report* 1986 16: 15–20. Jonathan Glover also argues that we owe children "a decent chance of a good life," though he does not explicitly claim this as a birthright for children. See Glover, *Choosing Children: Genes, Disability, and Design*, Oxford University Press, 2006.

Conversely, if parents cannot guarantee their children a life of minimal decency, whatever that might be, but are trying their hardest, may meet the minimal decency standard, and have few alternate routes to their own flourishing, maybe in some cases they should be permitted to risk procreation. Birthright principles are too rigid, making them unfair, and too vague, making them insufficiently action guiding.

In contrast, the principles I advocate are sensitive to parental circumstance and specific to procreative goods.

(ii) Non-Identity Problem Principles Few argue outright for non-identity principles of procreative permissibility, but many use the non-identity problem reasoning to set the standard of procreative care and, thereby, the principle of procreative permissibility, at a life worth living. According to this view, so long as a child's life is likely to be worth living, overall, procreation is permissible.[31]

There are numerous grave problems with this sort of principle. First, it's based on an ethical and metaphysical mistake because there really is no unsolvable non-identity problem (see Chapter 3). Second, even if we could not solve the non-identity problem, that does not mean that we should adopt its counterintuitive implications, which include permitting deliberately, negligently, and even maliciously inflicted disabilities and disadvantages, so long as the child's life is likely to be worth living, on balance. Parfit deemed the implications of the non-identity problem to be so counterintuitive that he thought they demanded of us an entirely new ethical theory—a theory that could avoid the non-identity problem's terribly counterintuitive implications.[32] A non-identity problem

---

31. See John Robertson, *Children of Choice: Freedom and the New Reproductive Technologies*, Princeton University Press, 1984.
32. Parfit, *Reasons and Persons*, 443.

principle is weighted entirely in favor of parental interests and not protective of children. It does not demand more of parents even when providing a higher level of procreative care would cost them next to nothing.

The principles I have argued for take children's interests into appropriate account and do not leave children having to content themselves with a life likely to be worth living, however barely, especially when better birth conditions would cost their parents little. Thus, they are more fair, more intuitive, and not based on ethical and metaphysical errors.

(iii) "The Best" or Eugenic Principles Some argue that one must create the "best" child that one can, in terms of the natural and social endowments the child will likely have.[33]

But this principle is too demanding of parents, requiring them to undergo significant, costly medical procedures, including in vitro fertilization, to test and screen embryos for various conditions so that they can select the "best" set of genes for their future child. Even for those who can afford the cost, it is very burdensome in terms of time and discomfort. It may also be less than best for children since it may undermine parental unconditional love by setting very high standards (the best!) for well-being. If you turn out grouchy, your parents have not received the best child (nor have you received the best temperament).[34] Finally, it assumes we have a settled account of what kind of life is "best," and that is likely too narrow a view of human well-being. A more moderate account of human well-being may make some claims, as I do,

---

33. See Julian Savulescu and Guy Kahane, "The Moral Obligation to Create Children with the Best Chance of the Best Life," *Bioethics* 2009 23: 274–290.
34. For a sustained argument against modern-day eugenics or seeking "the best," see Michael Sandel, *The Case against Perfection*, Harvard University Press, 2007.

regarding broad categories of human good, but demanding the "best" requires a detailed, specific, and comprehensive account of human good as well as a means of ranking all of those goods. That is a tall and unfilled order, and it is also not pluralistic regarding conceptions of the good.

Our principles, in contrast, allow for moderate pluralism regarding the good and, via the Motivation Restriction, protect unconditional love by building it into the permissible procreative motive. Our principles do not overly burden parents because parental burden is held in check by the requirement that it be justified by the stronger interest of the child in that case and context.

(iv) "Your Best" It might seem like common sense would tell us to just "do our best." How could we demand more of parents, and why would we ask for less for children? How can we hold anyone to a standard beyond their best—beyond what they can actually achieve? That seems clearly unfair and not action guiding. Therefore, "do your best" can seem like a reasonable and practical principle.

Except it's unfair to everyone. It is unfair to children because there are prospective parents whose procreative best is not good enough to meet children's basic needs. In such cases, procreation should probably not be permitted because it is irrational to run a very high risk of not having basic needs met at a very basic level for the benefit of being permitted to procreate under those kinds of circumstances. But "do your best" is unfair to parents as well. It is not always necessary and may well be extremely burdensome. In order for some people to really do their procreative best, significant sacrifices would have to be made in other important life areas, such as work or retirement savings, and if the child will be very well loved, raised, and nurtured with a lesser degree of parental sacrifice, there seems no clearly compelling reason to demand it.

The principles I advocate are more protective of children and more fair to parents as well.

(v) Procreative Liberty Principles Some argue for parental procreative liberty constrained only by the life-worth-living standard (to fall below that standard, on these sorts of accounts, is to harm the future child).[35] The claim is that procreating is central to identity and to one's personal values and is therefore a protected sphere of human freedom.

Of course, the problem with this view is that does not take children's interests into due account, and it justifies this flagrant injustice with non-identity problem reasoning that is deeply flawed.

Whereas procreative liberty principles are markedly one-sided, our principles aim for balance.

(vi) Strict Liability Seana Shiffrin argues in favor of a strict liability procreative standard for parents, a standard that will hold parents responsible for their children's procreative harms (very broadly delineated) and liable to demands for compensation.[36] As discussed in Chapter 4, Shiffrin holds all procreation to be seriously morally problematic due to the fact that children are created without their consent. Given this (alleged) rights violation

---

35. See John Robertson, "The Primacy of Procreative Liberty," in *Children of Choice: Freedom and the New Reproductive Technologies*, Princeton University Press, 1994; and "Procreative Liberty and Harm to Offspring in Assisted Reproduction," *American Journal of Law and Medicine* 2004 30: 7–40.
36. Seana Shiffrin, "Wrongful Life, Procreative Responsibility, and the Significance of Harm," *Legal Theory* 1999 5: 117–148.

and given life's precariousness, Shiffrin argues that procreation is unnecessary and extremely risky, like owning a pet lion. Therefore, the person who chooses to own the pet lion or to procreate assumes all responsibility for resulting harms, that is, strict liability.

The problem with procreative strict liability is that it misunderstands the nature and underestimates the significance of parental procreative interests. Procreating contributes uniquely to a person's social, spiritual, biological, and emotional life. There are many other ways to flourish but for those who want to procreate, not doing so incurs a steep and pervasive cost. It's not like owning a pet lion, which sounds like an ill-conceived, strange, and imprudent hobby. It is unfair to parents to classify their procreative interests as noncentral, easily replaceable by other interests, and not deserving of much respect or consideration. Strict liability is a one-sided procreative principle and, moreover, it ignores the many ways in which people create their own problems and difficulties once they are born. Not everything is your mother's fault.

The balanced nature of our principles stands in stark contrast to the one-sided strict liability principle.

(vii) Democratic Principles Some argue that procreation should be guided by principles of democracy and aimed at reducing oppression. In the procreative case, then, the goal would be to minimize intergenerational domination by restricting procreative intervention to only those that will enhance the future person's freedom from being dominated by others.[37]

---

37. See Anja J. Karnein, *A Theory of Unborn Life: From Abortion to Genetic Manipulation*, Oxford University Press, 2012, 87–91.

Although the goal of respect for the autonomy and independence of future persons is laudable, it seems ill fitting and uninformative to talk about domination in many common procreative contexts. Children should not be oppressed, of course, but talk of domination is not helpful when thinking about procreativity because children are not independent and their independent or autonomous wishes are largely unknown before they begin to develop as children and adolescents. Parents name and dress their children, decorate their bedrooms, choose their food, their language, and a good deal of their environment. Parents are in positions of great power over their children, and they must exercise their parental procreative role with due care to nurture their children's developing agency and autonomy, but it is not particularly clear or helpful to speak of avoiding procreative "intergenerational domination" when at least some degree of domination is unavoidable and a high level of paternalism is appropriate.

In contrast, our principles of procreative permissibility include self-respect (which requires a *self*; i.e., autonomy) and freedom from oppression as important procreative goods. Thus, parents are required to prioritize these goods for their children and nurture their child's sense of self, self-respect, and autonomy as developmentally appropriate. This seems like a more fitting way to protect future persons from domination than an unrealistic and unclear requirement to eliminate the dominance that parents naturally and, to a great extent, unavoidably have over their children.

(viii) Sanctity of Life/Gift Principles Some view all human life as sacred, valuable, worth living, and worth starting. This is usually a religious view that is part of a supernatural outlook. It is difficult to sustain a natural argument against a supernatural one. The two viewpoints talk past each other because they

differ in fundamental premises. I can only say what I have said at the outset. It seems incorrect to me to view life as a gift or as invariably worthwhile to the person living it. Moreover, there's a difference between claiming that all human life is worthy of respect for its own sake once it exists and the claim that any human life is worth creating. Of course we should treat everyone with respect, even people who are suffering from terrible diseases and disabilities. Suffering is a reason to help a person, not to disrespect her. That seems clear and uncontroversial. But there is no logic that requires us to connect these ideas of respect for persons with the claim that all lives are worth creating, regardless of how much the person living them is likely to suffer. As a procreative principle, sanctity of life protects children from some of the perils of a lack of unconditional love because it emphasizes the value of all persons for their own sake and regardless of any other factors. But it does not protect children from awful fates and severe suffering, from horrific diseases, disabilities, or abject poverty.

In contrast, our principles are consistent with respecting persons for their own sake and in their own right, but they also aim to protect children from being born into terribly adverse circumstance conducive to terrible suffering.

(ix) Who Needs a Principle? Many philosophers and bioethicists analyze procreative cases and issues on an ad hoc basis, with no clear commitment to any specified moral system or principle. The problem with that sort of approach to procreative ethics is that it is ad hoc and, as such, not particularly persuasive. Flying by the seat of one's intuitive pants from case to case is a chaotic fibrillation of inchoate values in need of systematic explanation and justification.

In contrast, our principles are systematic, based on well-established ethical theories, and supported by a consistent set of persuasive reasons. That gives us reason to think that we will usually be able to justifiably rely on them when we apply them to particular cases.

VII   FINALLY, TO THE CASES

A rule, as the saying goes, is only as good as the cases that make it up. Nowadays, it seems that some think that a rule is nothing *but* the cases, derived entirely from the results of case-based intuition contests and subject to change at the appearance of even one countercase. The Rawlsian view is that both cases and principles are important and relevant. It is also the moderate view (which has Aristotelian cachet). I have made my case for the principles I advocate. Now, let's look at some implications and applications of the principles.

Chapter 6

Procreative Principles in the Real World

I RECAP

We will now consider the implications and applications of our principles of procreative permissibility. They are:

The Motivation Restriction

Procreation must be motivated by the desire[1] and intention to raise, love, and nurture one's child once it is born.

Procreative Balance

Procreation is permissible when the risk you impose as a procreator on your children would not be irrational for you to accept as a condition of your own birth (assuming that you will exist), in exchange for the permission to procreate under these risk conditions.

Recall that due to the many rational approaches to risk, the term *irrational* is used here to mean that *everyone* has decisive

---

1. In order for the motivation to be appropriately reliable, desire must be present as well. A bare intent to raise, love, and nurture one's child once it's born, without the accompanying desire to do so, will not accomplish what the restriction is supposed to accomplish.

reasons against the act or decision in question (ceteris paribus). This is my definition of irrational (it is not identical to Rawls's use of the term), which I favor because it is both useful in drawing distinctions and reasonably pluralistic in its ability to accommodate the many rational approaches to risk. For example, although some may find behavior like hot-air ballooning irrational due to the risk versus benefit of this somewhat risky leisure activity, it would not be irrational for those who derive great joy from gliding to do so in this manner since the risk of a terrible outcome remains very low. It is not the case that everyone has decisive reasons against this act. So, for my purposes, the act would not be deemed irrational. In contrast, everyone has decisive reasons not to experiment with heroin since the costs can be extremely high and the benefits are not only dubious but also obtainable at far lesser levels of risk, with less addictive mind-altering drugs or nondrug experiences that confer similar benefits. Therefore, according to my analysis, experimenting with heroin is irrational, meaning, everyone has decisive reasons not to engage in that act.[2]

Procreative Balance is our central principle. The Motivation Restriction acts as a constraint. For those not persuaded by the Motivation Restriction, Procreative Balance can function on its own, without any additional constraints. Of course, I am persuaded by the Motivation Restriction and have tried to persuade you of it as well. Yet if I failed, there is still important action-guidance provided by the principle of Procreative Balance alone.

---

2. Exceptional cases will be exceptions to this general claim, e.g., there may be someone researching heroin addiction who has a compelling reason to try it under certain conditions, etc.

II PRELIMINARY IMPLICATIONS
OF THE PRINCIPLES OF PROCREATIVE
PERMISSIBILITY

Before we look at some paradigm cases, note that the principles of procreative permissibility have some illuminating and sometimes surprising implications:

(i) Procreative Diminishing Returns (aka Vindicated at Last: Your Parents Do Love Your Older Sister More Than They Love You) Most contemporary Western parents trot out the rote "I love all of my children equally," when pressed by their rivalrous children. The kids are not fooled. Parent-child relationships are not identical. Your first child makes you a parent and provides you with the opportunity to engage in the parent-child relationship as a parent. Your second child is just more of the same, baby. Harsh, but true. This does not mean that parents cannot love their second or fifth child just as much, or more, than their first. What it does mean is that the justification we have to procreate at all, namely, our deep and legitimate desire to be parents and raise children— to create a family—is, to a significant extent, exhausted by our first child. We have a weaker justification for creating a second child, and weaker still for a third, since we are by then parents twice over already. We may still have an interest in creating more than one child. Many think of a "family" as parent(s) and more than one child, for the parents' sake and the children's as well. Parents may enjoy parenting and want to engage in more of it. They may also enjoy the boisterous atmosphere of a larger family and mul- tiple family connections. Though there is no evidence that "only" children suffer much for their only-ness, siblings can be wonderful

lifelong friends and can help each other survive their parents' inevitable shortcomings. They can also be there for each other to share the burden of caring for aging parents. On the other hand, they can torment each other for life. Like most matters procreative, having multiple children is a risk but one that many find worth taking and worth imposing.

Procreative Balance tells us that as parental procreative interest decreases, procreative restriction increases because children's interests exert a greater pull on a lesser parental interest. We are seeking a balance of procreative interests. Picture a tug-of-war rope: the weaker the parental procreative liberty interest, the stronger the pull of the child's procreative goods interests. It's unlikely that Procreative Balance will ever permit procreating one's tenth child (barring special circumstances) because the parental interest in having ten rather than nine children is hardly significant and therefore too weak to counterbalance or outweigh the very significant risk of very significant suffering that all future children inevitably face by being thrust into life and the human condition.

Imagine parents whose children have a 1% risk of suffering from schizophrenia.[3] Schizophrenia involves terrifying psychotic hallucinations and delusions and interferes greatly with everyday functioning. It is also still very difficult to treat successfully.[4] We might think it acceptable for adults to procreate when their child has a 1% chance of developing schizophrenia. It is still a small

---

3. Although 1% is cited as the risk of schizophrenia for the general population, this does not differentiate between those with a family history of schizophrenia and those without. Since there is a strong genetic component to schizophrenia, the risk to the population without a family history of schizophrenia is less than 1%.

4. See Andrew Solomon, *Far from the Tree*, Scribner/Simon & Schuster, 2012, 295–353.

chance, and perhaps we can imagine accepting a small chance of a very horrible outcome for the benefit of procreative liberty. But would we think the same of the same couple imposing that same risk on their fifth child? Hardly. They have already exercised considerable procreative liberty; they have already reaped the benefits of engaging in the parent-child relationship as a parent. Their interest in having five children rather than four is too weak to justify procreating under a very small yet significant probability of a horrific outcome.

(ii) Disability or Discrimination? Nature or Nurture? Potato or Puhtahtoh? Bioethicists have spent considerable time, thought, and aggravation trying to figure out what a disability is.[5] Is it a natural or biological disadvantage, or is it a mere difference that becomes disadvantageous because society discriminates against it? Deafness is a paradigm case in this debate. Hearing is a natural ability that disadvantages those who lack it by making education, communication, and many professions difficult, but if sign language were widely spoken, being deaf would be far less disadvantageous and the claims of deafness as a culture rather than a disability would be more persuasive. Why, it may be argued, do we tell deaf people not to use preimplantation genetic diagnosis (PGD) to select a deaf embryo when we would never tell a mixed-race couple to use PGD to select their whitest embryo? These questions can make it seem important to

---

5. For an excellent collection of essays that capture the reasoning on both sides of this debate, see Kimberley Brownee and Adam Cureton, Eds., *Disability and Disadvantage*, Oxford University Press, 2009. For a sophisticated theoretical treatment of the debate, see Kristjana Kristiansen and Tom Shakespeare, Eds., *Arguing about Disability: Philosophical Perspectives*, Routledge, 2010.

determine whether disability is social, like illiteracy, or natural, like eye color.

But we will never know whether disability is a natural or social phenomenon because it's both. And one of the free gifts you get by signing on to the principle of Procreative Balance is that you can stop trying to solve the age-old unsolvable nature versus nurture mystery. Procreative Balance shows us that we don't have to answer this largely unanswerable question. A child is disadvantaged by being black in an apartheid society and deaf in a hearing society. How much of this burden is natural and how much is social does not matter much to the child and her ability to live a life of human flourishing. It is no comfort to be told that the fact that you can't communicate with the vast majority of the world's people is not due to your natural disability but is instead due to social discrimination. (If anything, that might make it feel a little worse because it then seems like the result of choice and human values rather than something that just unfortunately happened to happen.) Disadvantage is disadvantageous.

This, by itself, does not tell us which disadvantages we can permissibly risk for our children, but it does tell us that we need to focus on the parental interests and on the child and the life she will likely be able to lead rather than try to ponder or untangle the natural and cultural elements that factor into the bottom-line burden. Sidestepping the nature versus nurture disability debate doesn't mean that we will be insensitive to parental concerns. We can understand that parents may reasonably want children who don't tower over them—as in the case of achondroplastic adults—and also consider the disadvantage that being achondroplastic will be for their children. We can understand the burden born by African American children in the slave era (as did the

African American slaves, who often tried to terminate their pregnancies)[6] as well as the fact that having children may have been one of a precious few sources of happiness and meaning for slaves. What we have in this case is a tragic conflict of interests, not a conceptual problem about the nature of disability or disadvantage.

The principle of Procreative Balance helps direct our procreative ethics focus away from the disability debate morass and toward the practical and just adjudication of parental and child procreative interests. I consider this both a theoretical and a practical advantage of Procreative Balance. The theoretical advantage lies in showing us why and how we should avoid banging our heads against the unyielding wall of the nature versus nurture disability debate. The practical advantage is that by avoiding the "What is a disability?" question, we can focus on the interests of the people who matter and the circumstances that will impact their lives, regardless of how those circumstances are categorized.

(iii) Darwinian Cures When thinking about how Procreative Balance handles the procreative cases of carriers of genetic diseases or even the mildest of disadvantageous conditions, we may find ourselves tempted to "cure" these diseases and eliminate these disadvantages by banning their carriers from biological procreation. Since we are assuming that we will be born into and procreate under the principles we choose, it seems eminently rational of us to enact this sort of ban because then we thereby guarantee that we will neither suffer from nor carry the genes for these diseases

---

6. Elizabeth Fox-Genovese, *Within the Plantation Household: Black and White Women in the Old South,* University of North Carolina Press, 1988, 324.

or conditions. After all, if we ban all carriers of the color-blindness gene from procreating, when we are born under these rules we know that we will neither carry nor suffer from genetic color-blindness since anyone with those genes has been barred from procreating. Win-win for us, and we "cure" color-blindness in the bargain. A little too easy and probably unduly restrictive. (Isn't being banned from biological procreation worse than being color-blind?) What about those who carry or suffer from genetic diseases or disadvantageous conditions now? The contractualist thought experiment we are engaged in tells us to imagine that we could be anybody, and that assumption is key to the fairness of the principles we choose because it ensures that each person's interests are duly considered. But the prospect of Darwinian cures makes it seem like the interests of those who carry genes for genetic diseases but wish to procreate are not considered at all. We seem to be able to restrict their procreativity at no cost to ourselves, which circumvents the point of the veil of ignorance.

The solution to this Darwinian faux cure is the knowledge that we may remove our veils of ignorance only to discover that we have a genetic disease or carry a gene that will soon be discovered to be the marker of a genetic illness. It may not even be a very serious or disadvantageous disease, but now we can't procreate? Darwinian cures may also have societal implications that we may not want to endure. The fact that we may carry genes for genetic diseases and that the genetic causes of disadvantages and diseases are likely to continue to be discovered during our lifetimes forces us to consider the interests of those who carry the genes that cause diseases (and restores our confidence in the veil of ignorance). This does not mean that no carriers of genetic diseases will be barred from procreating. It just means that, instead of being cavalierly written off as a Darwinian win-win, the cost to the carriers of not procreating will be duly considered, as we consider the fact that we ourselves could be carriers of genetic disadvantage.

(iv) The Abortion Prize and Adoption Penalty Although I have made no claims regarding the moral permissibility of abortion or adoption,[7] their availability and permissibility impact applications of Procreative Balance. We tend to think of abortion as less than ideal and of adoption as a virtuous thing to do. Yet Procreative Balance awards a prize, of sorts, to those able to abort and penalizes those able to adopt. The abortion prize occurs because if a woman is able to screen for and abort a disadvantaged fetus, she will have greater procreative freedom in the many cases where fetal disadvantage increases with maternal age, for example. If you will screen for and abort a Down syndrome-affected fetus, you need not worry about postponing pregnancy for a few years (at least not on that account) because your delayed procreativity will not result in a person living with Down syndrome. If your fetus has Down syndrome, you will abort it. But if abortion is wrong and therefore you are unable to abort, you are obliged to worry about postponing pregnancy from thirty to thirty-five, say, because that delay exponentially increases the chances of your giving birth to a child with Down syndrome.[8] Procreative Balance may prohibit your delay. (If abortion is wrong and you are willing to abort anyway for the benefit of greater procreative liberty, then you get the sellout prize, I suppose.) Similarly, if you are able to adopt a

7. I refer here to the morality of adopting a child relinquished for adoption, not to the morality of choosing to relinquish a child for adoption.

8. At maternal age thirty-six, the risk of carrying a fetus with Down syndrome is one out of two hundred; at thirty-nine it is one out of one hundred. See Ernest B. Hook, Philip K. Cross, and Dina M. Schreinemachers, "Chromosomal Abnormality Rates at Amniocentesis and in Live-Born Infants," *Journal of the American Medical Association* 1983 249: 2034–2038.

child, then your interest in procreating a biological child is weaker than someone unable to adopt because restricting your biological procreation won't leave you with no opportunity to engage in the parent-child relationship as a parent. You will suffer the significant loss of biological procreation, but you will not suffer total procreative loss. Your interest in biological procreation is therefore weaker and thus subject to greater restriction than someone for whom adoption is not an option. For example, if your biological children will have a high risk of blindness and you can adopt children instead of procreating biologically, you lose less by being prohibited from biological procreativity than does a person whose biological children will have the same risk of blindness but who cannot adopt a child.

What kind of shoddy procreative principle rewards abortion and punishes adoption? Ours! Whoops. It looks like Procreative Balance has a deeply counterintuitive result. Is that a reason to reject the principle or to reject this implication? I don't think so.

Regarding adoption, it is simply true that procreative restriction has a much deeper and more pervasive impact on someone who can't adopt a child than it does on someone who can. Our principles should reflect this reality. This does not mean that someone can claim an ex post facto unwillingness to adopt just in order to gain greater biological procreative liberty. That sort of dishonest bargaining is in bad faith and not permitted by our contractualist framework. There are real obstacles to adoption and objective difficulties posed by adoption and the adoption process. Those are the difficulties that are countenanced by Procreative Balance. Recall that we apply Procreative Balance by asking ourselves if it would be irrational to accept the risk that our procreativity imposes on our future child as a condition of our own birth, in exchange for the permission to procreate under the risk conditions in question. The availability of adoption as an alternative is something we consider, not knowing our particular identity or our particular attitude toward adoption. What we consider about adoption is the range of rational attitudes we might turn out to have toward it. We can consider the money, time, effort, and heartache often involved in adoption. We can consider the biological loss, the worry about the lack of a biological connection, the lack of control over maternal behavior that can damage the fetus during pregnancy (e.g., fetal alcohol syndrome), and the increased possibility of a temperamental parent-child mismatch. Those are realities and, as such, ought to be considered. We also consider the positive realities of adopting a child, including, of course, the benefits of being able to engage in the parent-child relationship as a parent and the great altruistic feeling of raising a child already in existence and in need of parents. It is an advantage of Procreative Balance that these realities are taken into account even if the result (an adoption penalty, of sorts) may initially seem surprising. It is fair and reasonable to take into account the fact that prohibiting biological procreativity can sometimes be mitigated by adoption, but only when adoption is a viable option.[9]

Abortion, in this case, is not all that complicated. I do not take a position here on the moral status of a fetus and the morality of abortion. If abortion is permissible, then we sometimes have greater procreative leeway, as discussed. If it is not, then not. That seems correct. While an abortion prize, of sorts, seems counterintuitive, I suggest it is accurate to acknowledge that if abortion is indeed permissible, a wider array of procreative actions is available to us. It's actually not surprising that a greater degree of moral

---

9. Note that we already considered and rejected the possibility of requiring everyone to adopt rather than to procreate biologically. See Chapter 1.

choice allows for more permissible choices. Seen in this light, it makes sense that if abortion is permissible, we can take different and greater sorts of procreative risks since no child will bear their burden.

III   SOME PARADIGM CASES

Time to put the principles into real-world play. Let's look at some cases. Note that the cases are evaluated singly, assuming that the challenge addressed is the only one, for example, deafness or cystic fibrosis. Procreativity that involves multiple risks of multiple challenges to the child will have to be evaluated with all the risks considered jointly, making it less likely for procreation to be permissible in those cases.

(i) Natural Issues

a) *Genetic Diseases:* Many diseases are heritable, with known odds. Diseases that are autosomal recessive, meaning that it takes two copies of the abnormal gene for the disease to be present, are inherited at a rate of 25% if both parents carry the gene. If only one parent carries the gene, none of children will have the disease.[10] Tay-Sachs is an example of an autosomal

---

10. These are the most common scenarios for autosomal recessive diseases. If one parent has the disease and the other parent is a carrier, then 50% of their children will have the disease; if both parents are diseased, then all of their children will have the disease as well.

　　Passing a gene for a disease or disadvantageous condition to one's child may restrict the child's procreative liberty even if the child does not suffer from the disease or condition. The child is now a carrier and, as such, may be required to take care, in some instances, not to couple and procreate with another carrier of the same serious condition. I will not consider these sorts of disadvantages here as they are likely to be quite minor and the burden they impose is very difficult to ascertain. Most serious genetic diseases are fairly uncommon, since the worst and most common of them are the most likely to die out.

recessive genetic disease. Diseases that are autosomal dominant, meaning that it takes only one copy of the abnormal gene
for the disease to be present, are inherited at a rate of 50% if
one parent is diseased and at a rate of 75% if both parents are
diseased.[11] Huntington's disease is an example of an autosomal
dominant disease. There are also sex-linked genetic diseases,
in which the abnormal gene occurs on a sex chromosome, usually the X chromosome. Those diseases are more common in
boys since boys have only one copy of the X gene. Examples
of sex-linked genetic conditions include color-blindness and
hemophilia.[12]

On the more disadvantageous and less disadvantageous sides
of the spectrum, application of Procreative Balance is simple: Tay-
Sachs disease results in gradual loss of physical and mental abilities and death by age five. It is also painful. It is irrational to incur
a 25% risk of such a horrific outcome for the freedom to procreate
if you turn out to carry and partner with a carrier of the Tay-Sachs
gene. Indeed, since the availability of screening for carrying the
Tay-Sachs gene, the incidence of disease has plummeted as adults
who are coupled with other carriers of the abnormal gene refrain
from biological procreation, screen and abort affected fetuses,

---

11. These are the most common scenarios, assuming that the diseased parent has one abnormal
and one normal gene for the disease in question. If the diseased parent or parents have two
abnormal copies of the gene, then 100% of their children will be diseased.
12. The odds of sex-linked diseases are more complicated. For sex-linked recessive diseases, if
the mother is a carrier, then 50% of the sons and none of the daughters will be diseased. If
the mother is diseased, then all of the sons and none of the daughters will be diseased. If the
father is diseased and the mother is neither diseased nor a carrier, then none of the children
will be diseased. If the father is diseased and the mother is a carrier, then 50% of the children will be diseased; if the father is diseased and the mother is also diseased, then all of the
children will be diseased. For sex-linked dominant diseases, if the father is diseased, then
all of the daughters and none of the sons will be diseased. If the mother is diseased, 50% of
both daughters and sons will be diseased. If the mother is diseased and has two abnormal X
genes, then all of the children will be diseased.

or use PGD to screen out diseased embryos.[13] A far less burdensome genetic disadvantage (it doesn't merit the label "disease") is color-blindness. Color-blindness is a sex-linked recessive genetic abnormality. If a woman is color-blind, all of her children will be color-blind as well, but being color-blind does not have a very significant impact on one's ability to flourish. It is less than optimal health, I suppose, and it probably decreases one's ability to appreciate certain forms of art, but procreative restriction deprives people of a unique and deeply rewarding social connection (if one can adopt instead, one is still deprived of the biological connection to one's child and must also deal with the difficulties that often accompany the adoption process). Not being permitted to (biologically) procreate is not a small cost, and it is therefore rational to accept the risk, or the certainty, of being born color-blind in exchange for the liberty to procreate if one's children will be color-blind.

More complex cases include polydactyly, Huntington's disease, and cystic fibrosis. Polydactyly (being born with more than five fingers on each hand or five toes on each foot) is usually not very serious and does not impair human flourishing, though it can in more extreme cases. It can usually be treated with surgery. Given its limited impact on human flourishing, it seems rational to incur the risk of being born with polydactyly in exchange for the freedom to procreate biologically even though those born with polydactyly often require surgery. Huntington's disease is much more serious. If your parent has Huntington's, you have a 50% chance of developing the disease. It is a crippling disease that involves progressive physical and mental disability and is

13. Francis Collins, *The Language of Life: DNA and the Revolution in Personalized Medicine*, Harper, 2010.

eventually fatal, though many people with Huntington's die of suicide.[14] There is no treatment or cure. The rate of decline and age of onset of symptoms are determined by the extent of the genetic abnormality (specifically, by the number of abnormal CAG repeats on chromosome 4). Symptoms can begin in one's thirties or much later, depending on the severity of one's illness. Is it irrational to run a 50% risk of this awful and early pervasive mental and physical decline and death, if one's parent carries the Huntington's gene, in exchange for the freedom to procreate should you turn out to carry it? I think the balance here tips away from procreative freedom. Those born to a parent who suffers from Huntington's watch their parent's awful and inexorable total decline and disability, knowing that they have a fifty-fifty chance of suffering the same fate or worse (the number of abnormal CAG repeats tends to increase within families over time). Huntington's often cuts life off just as one's career and relationship efforts may be beginning to bear fruit and puts a stop to most forms of human flourishing. The possibility of using PGD to screen out embryos with the Huntington's gene further solidifies the case against procreative liberty (for those who will not use PGD) in this case.

Cystic fibrosis (CF) is an autosomal recessive genetic disease that affects the body's ability to regulate mucus, sweat, and digestive fluids. Life quality and lifespan for those with CF have improved significantly as better treatment options have been developed. Still, today, those with CF will suffer breathing difficulty, which can be extreme, recurrent sinus infections, and painful and constant treatments. Gastrointestinal and nutrition absorption difficulties are also common to CF, leading to liver disease (often

14. Medline Plus, "Huntington's Disease," web.

fatal), impaired growth, and diabetes. Infertility is common,[15] as is fatigue and incessant coughing. Mental function is not affected. Life expectancy with excellent medical treatment for children born with CF today is late thirties.[16] It's a pretty bad disease, yet those who suffer from it can still flourish in some respects because their mental and emotional abilities remain intact and they can function fairly normally, though this functioning is often interrupted by bouts of infection, fatigue, and illness. Is it irrational to risk being born with a 25% chance of having CF in exchange for the freedom to procreate as a carrier partnered with another carrier of CF? Here too, I think that the balance tips away from procreative liberty because CF's effects are so painful and pervasive, and a one in four chance is a very significant chance. And, even now when the life expectancy of someone with CF has increased so dramatically, it still leaves those with CF with, at best, half a life (and the knowledge of it). Is living without biological children less than half a life? Some might say so, and that's what makes CF a tough case. Here too the availability of PGD makes it much easier for me to say that for CF carriers PGD is required (so long as we find it permissible—more on that later). But even if PGD were not available, it seems an overstatement to say that a childless life is half a life. It can be if you leave the half that you would have filled with children empty, but you can choose to fill that half with other fulfilling relationships and pursuits. It will not be the same as having children and may well leave one with

---

15. The way we assess the procreative risk of infertility is the same way we assess any other procreative risk: just as we might consider whether it would be irrational to accept a 25% chance of being born deaf in exchange for the freedom to procreate if your children have a 25% chance of being deaf, we ask whether it would it be irrational to accept, say, a 50% chance of being infertile in exchange for the freedom to procreate if your procreativity imposes a 50% risk of infertility on your children.

16. Mayohealth.com.

a painful void, but one can still lead a life of human flourishing and achieve a high level of human goods. So I will bite the bullet: Procreative Balance rules against procreating without PGD for coupled carriers of CF.

b) *Genetic Predispositions to Physical and Mental Illness:* Nobody's perfect and we will all die of something. In many cases, knowing which diseases we are genetically predisposed to just tells us that we are more likely to die of cancer than of heart disease. But some of us are significantly predisposed to more serious ailments at a younger age. Breast, ovarian, and colon cancer risk can be inherited, and the risk can be very high,[17] but these cancers can also be treated, though with varying degrees of success, partially dependent on how early they are detected. For the most part, the inherited increase in risk is moderate (though it can sometimes be high, especially if predispositions are inherited from both parents) and can be mitigated by increased screening and prophylactic treatments, such as early colonoscopies with polyp removal for increased colon cancer risk and early mammograms or prophylactic mastectomy, ovary removal, or hysterectomy for increased breast, ovarian, and uterine cancer risk. These prophylactic treatments are invasive, painful, and anything but easy solutions to the problem of high cancer risk, but they may still teeter on the balance with procreative liberty, allowing procreators to proceed despite increased cancer risk to their children, since it seems quite possible to live a full and flourishing life and achieve high levels of most procreative goods despite the increased cancer risk. Exceptions will include possible cases of very high risk with lesser possibility of risk mitigation.

---

17. See http://cancer.stanford.edu/information/geneticsAndCancer/types/herbocs.html.

For most forms of mental illness, though the illness may be heritable to some degree, there are treatments that make a life of human flourishing possible. Currently, an exception is schizophrenia, which has serious and pervasive negative effects for which adequate treatments are still not available,[18] and it is not clear to what extent the risk can be mitigated. Schizophrenia is a brain disease that typically begins in early adulthood and devastates normal human thought, emotion, and expression.[19] It can make it impossible to achieve moderate levels of procreative goods such as health, social connection, education, self-respect, and even nourishment (because schizophrenia makes regular employment a rarity). Although schizophrenia has multiple genetic and environmental causes and triggers, it seems to have a strong heritable component, regardless of environment.[20] Having one parent with schizophrenia will confer at least a 10% risk of schizophrenia on the child.[21] Having two parents with schizophrenia results in a 40% risk of schizophrenia to the child.[22] A 40% chance of having a devastating chronic mental illness is clearly way more of an obstacle to having adequate levels of procreative goods and leading a life of human flourishing than is refraining from procreating if

18. In his well-researched book on difference, disability, and identity, Andrew Solomon singles out schizophrenia for its lack of a silver lining. Of persons with schizophrenia and their families, he says: "To me, their suffering seemed unending, and singularly fruitless." Solomon, *Far from the Tree*, 353.
19. See the *New York Times* In-Depth report on schizophrenia, web.
20. See R. Uher, "The Role of Genetic Variation in the Causation of Mental Illness: An Evolution-Informed Framework," *Mollecular Psychiatry* 2009 14: 1072–1082 and N. Craddock and I. Jones, "Genetics of Bipolar Disorder," *Journal of Medical Genetics* 1999 36: 585–594.
21. See Rebecca Frey, "Genetic Factors and Mental Disorders," *Encyclopedia of Mental Disorders*, web: http://www.minddisorders.com/Flu-Inv/Genetic-factors-and-mental-disorders.html. See also Johns Hopkins Health Library entry on schizophrenia: www.hopkinsmedicine.org/healthlibrary/conditions/mental_health_disorders/schizophrenia_85,P00762/.
22. See *New York Times* In-Depth report on schizophrenia, web.

you have schizophrenia and are partnered with someone who has schizophrenia. (The fact that two people with schizophrenia are unlikely to be able to provide adequate care for a child makes procreating in this sort of case even more morally problematic. Issues relating to parenting ability will be addressed shortly.) However, it is also irrational to accept a 10% risk of a completely devastating, lifelong, and incurable illness for the benefit of being able to procreate if you have that illness. Even though the odds greatly favor health—nine to one!—a 10% risk is quite significant, and schizophrenia is so pervasively damaging that it is an irrational risk to accept for the sake of being able to procreate biologically if one has schizophrenia. The rationality of accepting a risk depends on both the chances of a negative outcome and the nature of the outcome. In this case, because the negative outcome is so utterly devastating and the chances of it are quite significant, it seems irrational to accept the risk for the benefit of biological procreative liberty.[23]

c) *Disability:* First, a disclaimer: I am discussing disability in the section on natural issues because there is a natural component to disability. However, there is also a social component, and I will not attempt here to settle how much of disability is natural, how much social (as discussed earlier). Examples of disability include deafness, blindness, lack of mobility, and cognitive disability. Since one can still have a reasonable expectation of attaining a high level of procreative goods, if one has appropriate support in place, despite the

---

23. Because schizophrenia typically begins in early adulthood, just as parenthood becomes more of a real consideration to many people, it may be helpful in this case to consider whether a fertility treatment that had the side effect of causing schizophrenia in 10% of its recipients would be irrational to undergo. That is an irrational risk to take for the sake of its potential benefits. It certainly would not be a treatment that would survive medical regulation (it would be deemed not worth the risk).

challenge posed by a discrete noncognitive disability, Procreative Balance would seem to permit procreation in such cases, provided that parents are able and willing to help their children overcome their challenges. If one can adopt instead of procreate biologically, would Procreative Balance require that when there is a significant risk of a noncognitive disability? I am unsure of the answer in this case because there are so many variables, but, ultimately, I think the answer is likely to be no. Adoption is difficult, expensive, very often ultimately out of reach despite initial promise, and imposes the loss of a biological connection. That is no small set of parental losses, and it is unclear that risking a noncognitive disability demands that set of losses. I therefore don't think that Procreative Balance would demand adoption, when possible, instead of biological procreation when the risk of a noncognitive disability is present. There is room for reasonable disagreement here because there is more than one rational way to weigh the risk of noncognitive disability and the cost of adoption, but our principle tells us to rule in favor of procreative permissibility in that sort of case. In keeping with our broadly liberal values of autonomy and pluralism, when there are multiple rational approaches to risk, we err on the side of permissibility.

The (significant) risk of cognitive disability is different from physical disability because a significant cognitive disability will have a very significant negative effect on almost all procreative goods, except for the procreative good of not being oppressed. However, in many societies, cognitively disabled people are oppressed, and in most societies they are marginalized, which is a weaker form of oppression. Cognitive disability also restricts freedom, which is a form of oppression as well. It does seem irrational to accept a significant risk of a pervasive diminishment in one's ability to become educated (with all the opportunities for flourishing that entails), have deeper and more meaningful social connections, have a wide variety of sources of self-respect, and be in good health for the sake of permission to procreate biologically when your children would bear this sort of risk.

Multiple significant disabilities present a much greater challenge to procreative goods and to achievement of a life of human flourishing. Generally, it seems safe to say that it would be irrational to accept a significant risk of multiple significant disabilities for the sake of the freedom to procreate if your child would have a significant risk of multiple disabilities. However, in most cases of multiple significant disabilities, the risk is not known prior to the birth of the child and is often not genetic but the result of birth trauma or a nongenetic illness.

d) *Parental Age, Disease, Disability, Incompetence:* Parental age and disease can have effects on a child. Those effects are considered separately here, under their effects (e.g., if parental age results in an increased risk of cognitive disability to the child, it is discussed here under cognitive disability). Note that it will often be the case that in cases of people considering voluntary procreative delay due to career convenience or in order to increase financial security, the greater risk that delay will pose to the child's procreative goods will outweigh the parental procreative liberty benefit. This will be especially common when the delay involves postponing procreation beyond age thirty-five, when many serious procreative risks increase exponentially.[24] (The possibility and permissibility of

---

24. Down syndrome epitomizes this sort of risk, as discussed earlier (see Hook, Cross, and Schreinemachers, "Chromosomal Abnormality Rates"). The risks with increased maternal age are more known, but recent research has revealed significant risks of increased paternal age as well (see Brian M. D'Onofrio, Martin E. Rickert, et al., "Paternal Age at Childbearing and Offspring Psychiatric and Academic Morbidity," *JAMA Psychiatry*, online first, February 26, 2014, and Harry Fisch, Grace Hyun, et al., "The Influence of Paternal Age on Down Syndrome," *Journal of Urology* 2003 169: 2275–2278).

abortion or adoption will impact the way in which these risks play out as well, as discussed.) But parental age and disease may also affect a parent's ability to adequately raise a child. It is that issue I am addressing here. There may be some psychological adjustments that having a parent who has a disability or an illness may require of a child, but that does not, in and of itself, negatively impact the child's procreative goods or ability to lead a life of human flourishing. So long as parents are able to raise, nurture, and love their child, the parents' disease, age, or disability status per se is of no procreative relevance.

However, there are parental conditions that pose challenges to the ability to raise, nurture, and love one's child. The Motivation Restriction demands this intent of parents and the intent must be authentic, which, in turn, means it must be based on a reasonable and realistic ability to follow through on this intention for the duration of the child's childhood. People older than around fifty to fifty-five years old, say, are not in a position to claim that it is realistic to expect to be able to raise, nurture, and love their child to adulthood.[25] Although life expectancy in the developed world is beyond seventy to seventy-five years or so, most people do not persist much beyond their early seventies without health conditions that make sustained caretaking and childrearing unrealistic. This applies, of course, to men and women equally even though men are more commonly the ones procreating at older ages, given current

25. Having children when one is very young, e.g. a teenager, is an easy case because it poses risks to both the child and the teenager. Lose-lose; easy case. Having children earlier when delaying procreation would pose fewer risks to the child but would burden the parents is the kind of case that will be determined by the way in which the benefits and burdens stack up against each other in the particular case. If the risks posed to the child would be irrational to accept as conditions for one's own birth in exchange for the benefit to procreate under those risk conditions rather than delay, then the Balance Principle would require delaying procreation; if not, not.

biological constraints. We have many contemporary cases of men in their sixties or seventies having babies with younger women. Since the women are young enough to reasonably expect to live long enough to raise the children to adulthood, you might think it's okay for the men to be any age since the child will have a parent to raise her. But the Motivation Restriction does not permit this reasoning and, in my view, rightly so. For if the men in these cases cannot be said to be motivated by the desire to raise, nurture, and love their child (since it is not reasonable in these cases to expect to be able to raise the child to adulthood), what is motivating them to procreate? Candidates: vanity, enjoying being a parent while one can, pleasing a partner who wishes to have a child, deluding oneself about one's health and life expectancy, among others. These motivations fail to treat the child as a separate self, entitled to respect for her own sake. The Motivation Restriction applies to each person who is becoming a parent and incurring parental responsibility, and it demands the intent to raise, nurture, and love one's children throughout their childhood, not just for the first few years of it. One parent's failure to comply with it cannot be excused because the other parent is complying with it (even if we are talking about obligations to the same child—each parent is obligated separately).[26] This reasoning and restriction will also apply to people with a very significant risk of dying before their child reaches adulthood, due to their own health status, for example, having cancer with a poor prognosis.

---

26. We may wonder whether we can consider the couple as having a joint motivation or a "we intention" (see Raimo Tuomela and Kaarlo Miller, "We-Intentions," *Philosophical Studies* 1988 53: 367–389). I will not engage this debate here. To me, it is hard to imagine a joint motivation or intention as anything much more than two individual motivations or intentions that are similar in content. I don't see it as a way to share responsibility for motive or intent in any way that will allow one person to shoulder the motivational burden for another. But I flag this as a possible way for some to deal with this complex and counterintuitive case.

A strange and perhaps unacceptable result of the application of the Motivation Restriction to parental age is that a woman who might permissibly procreate when single (under certain conditions, as discussed in the next section) might be banned from procreating with her sixty-five-year-old husband since he, by virtue of age, is constrained from procreativity by the Motivation Restriction. Her husband, who will likely be a supportive presence in her child's life, at least for the first few years, acts here as a procreative barrier for her even though her children will be better, not worse off, for his presence. My view is that this result, though surprising, is correct. However, I can appreciate resistance to this conclusion because it is likely better, not worse, for the welfare of the child to have two parents, albeit one old for the job (or dead) than one. But the restriction here is a constraint demanded by respect, not by a straightforward welfare requirement, so it seems fitting to me that it sometimes operates in ways having no obvious or straightforward connection to welfare considerations. Those who find this result too contrary to common sense, everyone's best interests, and respectful treatment, can set this case aside as exceptional.[27]

Of course, there is no shortage of people who cannot reasonably expect to raise, nurture, and love their child because they just don't have nurturing or love in them, or because they have conditions that make it unlikely for them to be able to reliably and adequately raise a child. They are too angry, impatient, selfish, immature, superficial, mentally ill, cognitively disabled, or alcoholic to raise and nurture a child to adulthood. People with those sorts of challenges or proclivities may also fail to meet the requirements of

---

27. I say "straightforward" welfare considerations because the Motivation Restriction is, ultimately, good for us, in terms of our well-being. As argued, if we are not treated with respect and as ends in ourselves by parents, it will be difficult to develop a robust sense of self-respect, a vital and fundamental procreative good.

the Motivation Restriction, depending on the nature, severity, and incorrigibility of the difficulties in question. But let's not get carried away with this point. One need not be the kind of person who speaks in dulcet tones and reassures her child with "Good job!" for every trivial task accomplished in order to be deemed a reasonably loving, nurturing parent. Pluralism, my friends. Just as we accept all rational approaches to risk, we will accept all reasonably nurturing parenting styles and accommodate occasional nonhorrific lapses.

(ii) Social Issues

a) *Single Parenthood:* The research on the risks of being raised by a single parent is fraught with confounding variables that have proven nearly impossible to factor out. The most common problem associated with single parenthood is poverty. Impoverished people are more likely to become single parents in the first place, and single parents are at greater risk of becoming impoverished if they were not already. This makes the risks of being raised by a single parent extremely difficult to tease apart from the risks of being raised in poverty, but it also underscores how closely the risks are correlated. This is not surprising since two parents provide twice the income and nurturing opportunity for a child. Single-parent families are significantly more abusive, violent, and impoverished, and children in single-parent families are significantly less likely to achieve academic and social success.[28] Still, when poverty is

---

28. See Richard Gelles, "Child Abuse and Violence in Single-Parent Families: Parent Absence and Economic Deprivation," *American Journal of Orthopsychiatry* 1989 59: 492–501; W. H. Sack, R. Mason, and J. E. Higgins, "The Single-Parent Family and Abusive Child Punishment," *American Journal of Orthopsychiatry* 1985 55: 252–259; J. Belsky, "Parental and Nonparental Child Care and Children's Socioeconomic Development: A Decade in Review," *Journal of Marriage and the Family* 1990 52: 885–903.

factored out, these risks mostly fade to insignificance,[29] but since single parenthood is itself a contributor to poverty, it is not clear that the risks can accurately be teased apart completely. As boring as it may be, there is great advantage and security, with regard to most procreative goods, in doing things in the conventional order: adulthood, marriage, children.[30]

What can we make of these facts? All else being equal, it is less risky to a child's procreative goods to be born to two involved parents and, further, to parents married to each other. So I will stick my neck out here and say that if a couple remains unmarried because they find marriage a quaint, antiquated, irrelevant, or otherwise unattractive institution, it is important to note that marriage, generally, is protective of children[31] and, barring a very good reason, parents should marry for the sake of their children. Did I just say that? I believe I did. The facts generally support this general statement (which, like all general statements, will admit exceptions). However, if a single person is not at a significant risk for poverty even if she becomes a single parent, and she has ample social support, the risk posed to children being raised by a single parent may fade to the point that procreation may be permissible because the good of procreative

29. H. M. Blum, M. H. Boyle, and D. R. Offord, "Single Parent Families: Child Psychiatric Disorder and School Performance," *Journal of the American Academy of Child and Adolescent Psychiatry* 1998 27: 214–219; and Gelles, "Child Abuse and Violence," among others.

30. See Jason DeParle, "Two Classes, Divided by 'I Do,'" *New York Times*, July 14, 2012. This article draws on recent research that confirms the advantages of getting married before having children and some of the very significant risks of single parenting.

31. See Robin Fretwell Wilson, "Evaluating Marriage: Does Marriage Matter to the Nurturing of Children?" *San Diego Law Review* 2005 42. See also Maggie Gallagher, "What Is Marriage For? The Public Purposes of Marriage Law," *Louisiana Law Review* 2001–2002 62: 773–791. Note that the protective value of marriage for children is one (of many) reasons cited by gay activists in their fight for legal marriage equality.

liberty would outweigh the risk.[32] In states and countries where gay people are not permitted to marry, being a committed couple would likely do away with some of the risks associated with single parenting since the couple is only legally unmarried due to marriage discrimination.

b) *Poverty:* Poverty is bad for us. It eats away at all our procreative goods. It makes it difficult to maintain health, be well nourished, become educated, develop and maintain rewarding social connections,[33] have self-respect, and not be oppressed (since, in many societies, including the United States, those in poverty are marginalized and powerless, which is a form of oppression). I am speaking here about *abject* poverty: the inability to meet one's basic needs (e.g., food, shelter, and healthcare) at a basic level (i.e., at a level that allows you to avoid being malnourished, suffering from exposure, or suffering from an untreated treatable disease). It is irrational to accept a significant risk of abject poverty for the permission to procreate when one's children will be at risk of abject poverty. This is because abject poverty reduces most procreative goods to below threshold, minimal levels, and that has a deeper and more pervasively negative impact on procreative goods and the ability to achieve a life of human flourishing than procreative restriction does.

32. Numbers alone tell us that two parents are less risky for children than one (provided that neither parent is abusive). If you have two parents, you are less likely to have no live, employed, caring parents. These are risk factors crucial to child well-being that are cut in half by having two people raising a child rather than one.
33. Poverty makes it difficult to develop and maintain rewarding social connections because those who are in poverty are often working very many hours for whatever money they do have and therefore have less time to develop and maintain social connections. Poverty is also very stressful and alienating, often leading to depression, addictions, and other isolating behaviors. Furthermore, many ways of connecting socially cost money, e.g., sports, clubs, going out, etc.

If one's basic needs are met in a basic way, however, it is perhaps more challenging to achieve a life of human flourishing, but it may remain reasonably within reach so long as one remains somewhat autonomous and not oppressed. It does not seem irrational to risk being poor relative to one's society yet still have one's basic needs met at a basic level in exchange for the freedom to procreate and to exercise what may be one of your surest ways to flourish if you turn out to be one of the billions of people whose children run a significant risk of being poor.

Another procreative issue that arises in cases of the very poor is the age-old case of procreating in order to generate help on the family farm. Although this is not a case of poverty per se, it tends to arise under poverty or near-poverty parental conditions because otherwise, presumably, parents can pay someone to help them with their farming. It only makes sense to procreate only in order to generate help on the family farm if that help is needed to keep the farm going and the parents cannot afford to pay for it. So, instead, they create it and generate free help. This free help has to be fed but not paid beyond basic nourishment. Clearly, if parents are really having a child just in order to generate free labor, that violates the Motivation Restriction and is impermissible. If it was ever truly a common practice, so much the worse for what used to be a common practice. Historically, slavery was common too, and this sort of procreativity does not seem so very different in spirit. As noted, however, procreation can be multiply motivated. So long as the desire to raise, love, and nurture the child is present and prominent, other motivations may be permissible as well.

c) *Oppression:* Oppression comes in many varieties and intensities and can be more or less of a challenge to procreative goods and a life of human flourishing. It is also extremely common. Most of the world is sexist, racism remains commonplace, in many parts of the world anti-Semitism has practically reverted to respectability, and homophobia is widespread. In many cases where a child will likely be oppressed to some degree, the nature and degree of the oppression are less of a threat to procreative goods and a life of human flourishing than procreative restriction (which can also be somewhat oppressive) would be. In those cases, the presence of oppression would not make procreation impermissible.

Unfortunately, there are many cases of oppression where the risk to the child's procreative goods seems greater than the risk that procreative restriction would pose to parental procreative goods. Yet, even in such cases, it may be too quick to simply say that procreation is prohibited by Procreative Balance. There are several factors that complicate evaluating procreation when oppression threatens. For one thing, in many cases of severe oppression, prospective parents have little procreative control. Sometimes not procreating would imperil their lives and then the balance of benefits and burdens would likely tip in the parental direction unless the child's life was likely to be not worth living, or even worse than death. If one's child's life was likely not to be worth living, yet not procreating may well get you killed, the scale might hover in balance, unable to tip toward either side. I am not sure that we can demand that people die in order to spare their children a fate worse than death because I am not sure that self-sacrifice is something that can be demanded of people even if it would be the best thing to do. It may simply be too much to ask of anyone, given the biological and psychological drive to self-preservation. There may also be cases where procreative restriction would require that couples refrain from intercourse, further burdening an already oppressed couple and depriving them of an important aspect of human relationships and a unique source of intimacy. To justify that sort of deprivation via Procreative Balance, the oppressive threat to the child would have to entail a life more deprived still. Finally, there is the special burden imposed by demanding that oppressed people participate in their own annihilation or genocide by letting themselves die out. That is quite the twist of the knife and counts against procreative restriction. But only up to a point: it counts as a burden to the parents, thereby making procreative restriction less likely due to Procreative Balance, but it does not allow us to override the Motivation Restriction and procreate solely or primarily as a means of ensuring group continuity (because that treats the child as a mere means for the good of the group rather than as a separate self, entitled to respect as an end in herself).

That is no small list of complications. One thing that reduces the difficulty of figuring out what is permissible in these cases is the fact that parents whose children risk severe oppression are less likely to want to procreate because they won't want to put themselves or their children through that sort of ordeal. But this uncomplicating factor may not be present, for example, in severely sexist societies, where one or even both parents see the sexism as a valued religious or cultural practice.[34]

We may still ask how our principles direct those who can avoid procreating and whose children risk severe oppression. Let

---

34. I will not engage here in a debate about cultural relativism, as I have already argued for a universalistic set of human goods (see Chapter 5). It is bad for people to be oppressed. The relativistic controversy is about what counts as oppression, not whether it is bad for people. Some may argue that sexism is, in many cases, cultural, not oppressive, and should be tolerated. I reject this view, as do many of the women living in sexist cultures, but I do not argue the point here. For discussions regarding this controversy, see Seyla Benhabib, "Cultural Complexity, Moral Interdependence, and the Global Dialogical Community," in Jonathan Glover and Martha Nussbaum, Eds., *Women, Culture, and Development*, Oxford University Press, 1995, 235–255.

us look at the cases of American slavery, the Holocaust, the Taliban regime in Afghanistan, and sexism in Saudi Arabia. Imagine an African American slave in the Deep South. Her child will be born into slavery, not allowed to go to school or learn to read, may well be malnourished, will likely be beaten, humiliated, have no autonomy or freedom, and be treated as property, making self-respect very difficult to achieve and maintain. The child is also at risk of being sold away from her parents or loved ones at any point and can be (legally) raped by her owner.[35] It seems irrational to accept a near certainty of being born into these conditions for the freedom to procreate under these conditions. On the other hand, how can we say to those who are living such an oppressed life already, and suffering such unfathomable human injustice, "No kids (or intercourse) for you!" I am not sure that we can, even though I think that not procreating would be the right thing to do under the circumstances. Circumstances this tragic make it difficult, and perhaps wrong, to hold people accountable for their irrationality.

The Holocaust is a simpler case because the threat of extreme torture and death for Jews under Nazi control was so immediate and extreme.[36] What would be the point of procreating under those sorts of conditions? Your baby is slated for a short painful life and a painful death, if you defy the odds and live to give birth to her. The fact that the Holocaust occurred during a war that was

---

35. These facts about life as an American slave are well documented and well known. See Frederick Douglass, *Narrative of the Life of Frederick Douglass*, Bedford/St. Martin's, 2002; and *Born in Slavery: Slave Narratives from the Federal Writer's Project, 1936–1938*, Library of Congress, http://memory.loc.gov/ammem/snhtml/snhome.html, among many others.
36. These facts about the Holocaust are well documented and well known. See Claude Lanzmann, director, *Shoah*, 1985; The University of Southern California Shoah Foundation archives, http://sfi.usc.edu/; and Lucy Davidowitz, *The War against the Jews: 1933–1945*, Bantam, 1975, among many others.

expected to end eventually further confirms the rationality of forgoing procreation as a European Jew during the Holocaust since one might hope to procreate when the murderous regime ended (if one survived, which was exceedingly unlikely).

Procreation under the influence of the Taliban regime in Afghanistan is quite complex because the sexist oppression is extreme and the extent and duration of the Taliban's control are changing and unknown. At some points under Taliban rule, women were barred from employment, education, all forms of public life, and all forms of dress with the exception of the burka.[37] Here too, it seems irrational to accept the high risk (around 50%) of being born into severely oppressive conditions for the freedom to procreate under severely oppressive conditions. Perhaps the refusal to procreate will itself serve as a protest and help inspire change. Sadly, this discussion is mostly moot since there is such a low level of procreative liberty in Afghanistan that it seems nearly pointless to say that Afghan adults should choose not to procreate under the Taliban regime. Nevertheless, I believe that is what they ought to choose, if possible, because it is irrational to risk that sort of oppressed life for the freedom to procreate under those risk conditions.[38]

On the other hand, if all justice-minded, moral people choose not to procreate, who will lead the revolution and press for change? Perhaps this is a case where third-party interests should be considered but are not, due the limitations of our inquiry (we are

37. See Vincent Iacopino, "The Taliban's War on Women," report for Physicians for Human Rights, http://physiciansforhumanrights.org/library/reports/talibans-war-on-women-1998.html and Rosemarie Skaine, *The Women of Afghanistan under the Taliban*, McFarland, 2002.

38. The risk is very high since about 50% of children are born female. Furthermore, it is not good for men to participate in sexist oppression either as it distorts their relationships, depriving them of true companionship and intimacy with the women in their lives.

considering only the interests of prospective parents and their future children). However, I think that the Motivation Restriction withstands the pull of the possible third-party interests here since it seems to me that we may not create people solely or primarily for the good or purposes of others, even third-party others. Creating a child solely or primarily to suffer for the sake of others seems like exactly the sort of case the Motivation Restriction is intended to prohibit.

Consider the case of sexist oppression in Saudi Arabia: Imagine the change that might be possible if Saudi Arabian citizens did what they could to avoid procreating due to the severely oppressive sexism that currently prevails. It would be a powerful protest statement. Today, every Saudi woman must have a male guardian whose permission is required for her to marry, divorce (tricky since the guardian is often her husband), go to school, work, have elective surgery, or travel if she is younger than forty-five. Saudi women may only work in environments where they serve women only. They cannot vote or drive and must cover most of their bodies when outside with a burka or abaya. Their legal testimony is equivalent to that of half of a man's, and rape victims are often punished by the legal system, society, and their families (for dishonoring the family).[39] Women in Saudi Arabia have little autonomy and few adult rights. Is it irrational to accept the very high risk (around 50%) of being born into such oppressive conditions as a Saudi girl for the benefit of freedom to procreate under such conditions as a Saudi adult? It

39. These facts are widely acknowledged to be true and are not disputed by Saudi authorities. See Wikipedia entry on "Women's Rights in Saudi Arabia," web. See also Adam Coogle, "Saudi Arabia to Women: 'Don't Speak Up, We Know What's Best for You,'" *Daily Beast* and Human Rights Watch, June 26, 2013, http://www.hrw.org/news/2013/06/26/ saudi-arabia-women-dont-speak-we-know-whats-best-you.

seems irrational. Not procreating removes one very important and unique relationship and pursuit from one's life. It's a significant loss and reduces one's capacity to flourish. But being so globally controlled and being deprived of autonomy in marriage (in both marital status and spousal choice), education, and employment has a more pervasive negative effect on one's procreative goods and ability to lead a life of human flourishing. I conclude that since the oppression in Saudi Arabia is so pervasive and severe, procreativity is prohibited by Procreative Balance when complying with this prohibition would not imperil life or health.

(iii) Reproductive Technologies

a) *IVF, ICSI, and WCN (Whatever Comes Next):* Some reproductive technologies that were once controversial have become largely accepted today. In vitro fertilization (IVF), or "test-tube babies," is an example of such technology. At its introduction, people worried about overriding nature and playing god, but we hear little about these worries today. More recently, yet without much fanfare, intracytoplasmic sperm injection (ICSI), where a single sperm is injected into an egg to facilitate fertilization in the course of an IVF procedure, became an accepted treatment for certain forms of infertility. Currently, cloning is a developing technology that might have reproductive applications. The worry I have regarding new reproductive technologies and techniques is that they are, when new, experimental. Experimenting on children for the sake of their parents is problematic because parental consent on behalf of the child is undermined by the conflict of interests in these kinds of cases, resulting in experimenting on human subjects with questionable consent. But it is not clear to me what risks are involved and if they rise to the level that

Procreative Balance might prohibit.[40] (Of course, the Motivation Restriction might prohibit some uses of WCN, depending on the motivation for their use.) I raise this as a procreative problem for further thought.

b) *Preimplantation Genetic Diagnosis (PGD):* PGD involves testing embryos for specific genetic markers or patterns and then selecting embryos for implantation, based on the results. It is used, generally, to screen for serious diseases with known genetic markers, such as cystic fibrosis or Tay-Sachs. It is also used for sex selection.[41] In order to isolate and test embryos before they are implanted and develop in utero, IVF is required. This makes PGD an expensive, difficult, and often uncomfortable process.

We may wonder whether PGD is permissible. If we find it permissible, we may then wonder whether it is ever or often required. We may, of course, find it impermissible.

• *Permitted or banned:* Why not PGD? PGD can enable couples and children to avoid suffering from Tay-Sachs, cystic fibrosis, or femaleness. It can allow couples to makes sure that their children will not have Fanconi anemia, Marfan syndrome, or the ability to hear (some deaf couples have a very strong preference for a deaf child). It is permitted to use PGD at least in some instances, for example, to prevent the birth of a child with a life

---

40. IVF involves multiple strong hormonal medications for the mother with effects not entirely known. The effects of IVF and ICSI on children are unknown as well. A recent study concluded that children born of IVF have higher rates of learning disabilities and autism, though the risk remains very, very small. See Kate Kelland, "Some Forms of IVF Linked to Rise of Autism, Mental Disability," Reuters International, July 2, 2013.

41. See Molina B. Dayal, Richard Scott Lucidi, et al., "Preimplantation Genetic Diagnosis," *Medscape Reference*, August 29, 2011, http://emedicine.medscape.com/article/273415-overview#aw2aab6b4.

not worth living. There does not seem to be a compelling reason to ban PGD entirely, especially since it can sometimes allow prospective parents to permissibly procreate by enabling them to screen out embryos that they would not normally be permitted to risk procreating (e.g., embryos with Tay-Sachs disease or anencephaly). On the other hand, using PGD to select for the embryo with the bluest eye or maleness seems impermissible.

It is common for people to think that it is a good idea to use PGD to select against embryos slated for serious diseases or disabilities but not to select in favor of disability or for specific traits not associated with health or disease, for example, sex, hair color, or athletic ability. I suspect that the common view is onto something. But a consistent set of persuasive reasons for this common view has yet to be articulated. I will try to do that now.

We can distinguish between using PGD to select for traits directly related to the child's well-being and using PGD to select for traits that are only indirectly related to the child's well-being or largely irrelevant to the child's well-being, but preferred by the parents. It is instructive to consider the motive for screening. Are we selecting for or against characteristics that are important to the child's natural ability to enjoy procreative goods and live a life of human flourishing? Those sorts of choices are in keeping with our concern for a child's well-being and seem, for the most part, unobjectionable. We may wish to avoid creating a child that will face significant challenges to well-being when we can, instead, create a child with fewer (known) challenges to living a life of human flourishing. But when we select for gender or in favor of deafness, we seem to be making this choice primarily for ourselves, so that we get the kind of child we want. If we think that we will not be able to love a girl as much as a boy or communicate with a hearing child as well as we could communicate with a deaf child, those considerations are not directly for the child's sake. They are only arguably for the child's sake indirectly, because of our own preferences and proclivities. If we allow for that indirect view of what we are doing to count as acting for our child's sake, we can smuggle in almost any act just by claiming that we will treat the child better if we are permitted to do what we want. We can even intend to beat the child moderately because if we are not permitted that outlet for our violent enjoyments, we will be unable to control ourselves and beat the child severely and mercilessly. But that is clearly not what it means to do something for someone *else*'s sake. In order to claim to be acting for the child's sake, we must be acting for the child's sake directly, and not derivatively or indirectly.

Tailoring your child, not directly for her sake, but, instead, to suit your preferences and proclivities bespeaks a lack of unconditional love and demonstrates an attitude inconsistent with treating a child as an end in herself.[42] Being a parent requires the intention to love unconditionally, for the child's sake, because that is what children need (see Chapter 2), and it is also paradigmatic of the uniqueness of the parent-child relationship, which is ostensibly what you are after as a parent in compliance with the Motivation Restriction. Using PGD to screen out traits that you, as a parent, would prefer your child not to have for your

---

42. See Michael Sandel, *The Case against Perfection: Ethics in the Age of Genetic Engineering*, Harvard University Press, 2007. He says: "The problem [with genetic enhancement] lies in the hubris of the designing parents in their drive to master the mystery of birth. Even if this disposition does not make the parents tyrants to their children, it disfigures the relationship between parent and child, and deprives the parent of the humility and enlarged human sympathies that an openness to the unbidden can cultivate" (46). For a reply to Sandel, see David DeGrazia, *Creation Ethics: Reproduction, Genetics, and Quality of Life*, Oxford University Press, 2012, 128–129.

own sake displays attitudes inconsistent with the Motivation Restriction.

However, we may still ask what makes it okay to use PGD to select for the child who can hear, which is likely to create a child with fewer (known) challenges to well-being, but not for the child with the most beautiful eyes or the whitest skin, which often is also thought likely to create a child with fewer (known) challenges to well-being. These possible uses of PGD may be undertaken for the child's sake, in order to increase the odds of having a child with a high level of well-being, yet they don't avoid disease or disability. So why object to using PGD in those cases?

Three reasons: First, some of the traits we are talking about are easier to live without only because people who have them are discriminated against in our society. If we are using PGD because we too value people with darker skin less than people with lighter skin, then we are directly participating in racism, and that is wrong for the same reasons that racism is wrong. Similarly, to use PGD to select for gender because we value one gender over the other is to participate in sexism and is wrong for the same reasons that sexism is wrong. To use PGD to select for gender because we buy into sexist preconceptions about gender differences is also to participate in sexism and is similarly wrong.[43]

Yet we can easily imagine parents who may wish to use PGD to select for traits that are easier to live with only due to social discrimination, not because the parents are bigoted but because they

---

43. I make no exception for cases of so-called "family balancing" wherein gender selection is done only by parents who already have a child, or children, of one gender and wish to experience parenting a child of the other gender. To assume that parenting differs so importantly by gender rather than by the actual child one parents is sexist. As a woman married to a man and the parent of two boys, I never found my family gender imbalanced and I am not sure that is even a coherent notion (are we going to topple over from an excess of the Y chromosome?).

wish to shield their child from prejudice. That sort of use of PGD would be directly for the child's sake, yet it would still be an act of participation in sexism or racism in that it would be an instance of disvaluing a trait that should not be disvalued on its own terms (for what it is). By selecting for gender or race, over time, we may make sexism and racism seem natural and inevitable—see? everyone who can afford it screens out the girls and the nappy hair! This can have the unintended effect of helping to entrench or seeming to endorse discrimination. This does not seem like the best way to ease your child's life, because prejudice is a societal scourge and, as such, is not good for anyone. The more we can combat or undermine it rather than perpetuate or participate in it, the better it is for everyone, including the child.

Imagine a cosmetic surgical procedure that costs a lot of money but could successfully lighten a person's skin tone. If parents subjected their child to that sort of surgery just to make life a little easier, that does smack of racism, even if the parents are not motivated by racism, and it may also serve to perpetuate racist attitudes and values (e.g., dark skin is undesirable, bad, unattractive, etc.). This does not mean it would never be permissible. In cases of extreme racism, it may be necessary for a child's welfare to undergo such a surgery, and in extreme circumstances like that, it would similarly be permissible to use PGD for the same purposes (especially since in the absence of PGD, procreation might be impermissible, depending on the severity of the prevailing racism).

Some might argue that some disabilities, for example, deafness, are only disadvantageous due to societal discrimination. This is an exaggeration. Just because it would be far less disadvantageous to be deaf if more people spoke sign language, that does not mean that the disadvantage of deafness is *entirely* societal. There is a natural aspect to the disadvantage of deafness: deaf people cannot hear danger, music, or the human voice. We need not tease apart how much of the disadvantage of disability is natural or environmental here because I am only arguing that PGD is usually impermissible when used to select against traits that are only disadvantageous due to societal discrimination, that is, traits that are not naturally disadvantageous at all. Exceptions, as discussed, will include cases of using PGD to protect one's children from severe prejudice.

The second reason to object to use of PGD to screen for the whitest skin, the bluest eye, or musical ability is that focusing, allegedly for the child's sake, on specific traits not associated with disease or health is a misguided approach to human well-being. Although it is often considered desirable to be tall, athletic, attractive, and of superior intelligence, it is not the case that people with these traits are more capable of enjoying procreative goods and living a life of human flourishing than those with different traits. There are multiple paths to flourishing and multiple ways to flourish. Blondes may have more fun, but they are not more capable of human flourishing, generally, nor are fast runners or mathematicians. To select for specific traits not associated with disease or health makes a mistake about human well-being and models mistaken values for one's children and, in that way, sets them up for failure. If our children think that their chance at a life of human flourishing depends to any serious extent on their ability to engage or excel in sports, math, music, modeling, or any one specific trait, talent, or pursuit, they are missing out on the richness and reduced anxiety available to those who realize that there are many ways to flourish. Broad and significant avenues of human flourishing, like social connections and opportunities for expressions of creativity, are important for human well-being, and if we could use PGD to secure them, we might have good reason to do so, but that is consistent with using PGD for traits associated with disease or health since the inability to have deep social connection or to express creativity is not the normal, healthy human state.

The third reason to object to using PGD to select for traits not significantly associated with disease or health (conditions that significantly affect the ability to live a life of human flourishing) is that it is bad parenting; bad for children and bad for parents. It is too controlling and displays an unrealistic and inappropriate attitude about parental influence. You can't make your child's life go as planned, down to the color of her eyes or her ability to excel in soccer or math. Your child may indeed have the mathematical or musical ability you use PGD to select for, but that doesn't mean she will excel at math or music, and, more importantly, it doesn't mean that she will be any more likely to lead a life of human flourishing. Maybe she will be a very miserable and lonely genius. Maybe she will become a clown or a drug addict instead of a concert pianist. Parents would do better by their children (and themselves) in terms of procreative goods and leading a life of human flourishing by nurturing their children's autonomy and resilience than by trying to micromanage their lives, down to the color of their eyes or their ability to run very fast.[44]

For these reasons, using PGD to screen out embryos with significant natural barriers to living a life of human flourishing, for example, deafness, Tay-Sachs, cystic fibrosis, or mental retardation, is permitted. Using PGD to screen for traits not broadly significant to living a life of human flourishing, for example, height,

44. This is an empirical claim. For empirical support for this claim, see Holly H. Schiffrin, Miriam Liss, et al., "Helping or Hovering? The Effects of Helicopter Parenting on College Students' Well-Being," *Journal of Child and Family Studies*, February 9, 2013; Terri LeMoyne and Tom Buchanan, "Does Hovering Matter? Helicopter Parenting and Its Effect on Well-Being," *Sociological Spectrum* 2011 31: 399–418; and Eli J. Finkel and Grainne M. Fitzsimons, "When Helping Hurts," *New York Times*, May 10, 2013, among many others.

athleticism, or musical ability, is probably not. And, just as sexism and racism are impermissible in other areas of human activity, it is not permissible to use PGD to participate in wrongful discrimination. It is problematic to use PGD to protect one's child from mild to moderate prejudice, but it is permissible to use PGD when needed to shield a child from extreme prejudice.

Savior siblings: I will discuss savior sibling cases in the context of PGD because when people decide to procreate to generate body parts or products for their existing sick child, they now usually use PGD to do so because that can sometimes ensure that the child they create has body parts and products compatible with those of their existing sick child. Note, however, that savior sibling cases preceded the availability of PGD. Before PGD was available, people would sometimes create siblings naturally for their existing sick child in the hopes that their new child would be born with body parts and products compatible with those of their existing sick child. Savior siblings are controversial because creating them may violate the Motivation Restriction. Parents who procreated savior siblings have been accused of using their younger child as a mere means for the preservation of their older child. This is not, in my view, an entirely unreasonable view of what sometimes happens in these kinds of cases.[45] If the only reason you are creating a new child is because this is your surest way of saving your existing child, that procreativity violates the Motivation Restriction—it does not treat the child as a separate self, entitled to respect for her own sake.

45. Example of an off-putting savior sibling scenario: imagine a couple who cannot use PGD to select a body part/product-compatible savior sibling embryo, so they decide to take their chances with a natural pregnancy. They get pregnant, test the fetus in utero for compatibility, and abort it if it is not compatible with the existing sick child. This has happened. (See Lisa Belkin, "The Made-to-Order Savior," *New York Times*, July 1, 2001.)

However, what sometimes (perhaps often) happens in these cases is that the parents of the sick child consider having another child in order to save the first child and then become genuinely interested in and committed to the idea of having the additional child, for its own sake as well as for the sake of their older, sick child. Because procreative motivation is complex and can be multiply motivated, it is possible that some savior sibling cases are permissible. My suspicion is that sometimes parents of savior siblings are initially wholly motivated by the desire to save their existing child. But they cannot really stomach having a child solely for the use of another child and they also, once they begin to think about creating another child and engage with that idea, begin to see the future child as a real person and a real child of theirs, and the more acceptable procreative motivation then kicks in. If my speculation is correct, then those sorts of savior sibling cases are permissible. There are also cases where parents of a sick child had always intended to have another child but had not yet done so, for whatever reason, and choose to proceed with conception in time to possibly give birth to not only the additional child they had always wanted but also to a child that can possibly save their sick child. This sort of case does not seem to violate the Motivation Restriction either. (It would be perverse and unjustified to ban procreation to parents who would otherwise be permitted to procreate, just because doing so might create a bone marrow donor for their existing sick child.)

Using PGD to select for an embryo with body parts and products compatible with saving the existing child rather than procreating naturally, partially in hopes for a savior sibling, may seem permissible whenever creating a savior sibling is permissible, since it is done to save a life and does not seem to harm the future child.[46] However, it is a case of using PGD to select a trait that is not selected for the child's sake. It is selected for a different child's sake, that is, the existing sick sibling. If it is not permissible to use PGD to select for traits for the parents' sake, why might it be permissible to use PGD to select for a trait for a different child's sake? On the other hand, imagine parents who are having the second child they had always planned for and always wanted, and who can use PGD to save their existing sick child, but forgo the technology so as not to select a trait that is not selected for the sake of the child who will have that trait. That does not seem to value the first child properly since it passes on a chance to save that first child's life in a way that would likely not harm anyone else. All parties involved have reason to accept PGD in this sort of case: the parents want to save their sick child, the sick child wants to be saved, and the future sibling would likely grow up to be proud to have helped save her sibling. Contractualism seems to argue for acceptance of PGD in these kinds of cases; if we did not know who we would turn out to be, we would want to allow PGD in these kinds of cases to further our legitimate interests. Yet the application of our principles to savior sibling cases would seem to ban the use of PGD in these cases for the same reason it would ban deaf parents from using PGD to select a deaf child: it is not a trait selected for the sake of the child.

I believe that this is a case where third-party interests play a vital role that is not considered by our principles. Our principles of procreative permissibility are designed to take only

---

46. Because using PGD to select savior siblings is a relatively new technology, we do not yet have a population of savior siblings to study for adverse effects of the way in which they were conceived. However, if they were conceived in compliance with our procreative principles, we don't have reason to think that they will be harmed by the way in which they were conceived (or the reasons for which they were conceived).

the interests of the parents and the future child into account. They are therefore limited in cases where third-party interests properly play a significant role. The sick sibling is a third party not given due consideration here by our limited principles. If that sick sibling can be saved by using PGD to select a compatible donor sibling, in cases where parents are not in violation of the Motivation Restriction by having another child, it seems to me that due consideration of the sick child permits use of PGD to select a compatible donor sibling. Although selecting a savoir sibling is not done for the sake of the savior sibling directly, it is consistent with the savior siblings' interests because, barring unusual circumstances, most people would want to save their sibling's life. This fact adds to the case in favor of allowing PGD in savior sibling cases that do not otherwise violate our principles.

• **Required:** When permissible, is PGD required? It is required when not using PGD would render procreation impermissible, for example, in cases of partnered carriers of Tay-Sachs disease. It may also be required when use of PGD would result in greater child benefit than parental detriment (in keeping with Procreative Balance). But since PGD is currently very expensive and uncomfortable, it is unlikely to be required except to screen out embryos with extremely disabling or painful conditions.

c) *Sperm/Egg Donation:* If sperm and egg donors and sellers are parents, as argued in Chapter 2, then they are parentally responsible and required to comply with our procreative principles. Because gamete donors/sellers do not intend to raise, love, and nurture their children to adulthood, they are in violation of the Motivation Restriction. Gamete donation or sale is, therefore, not permitted. (For those not persuaded by Chapter 2's argument that gamete donors are parents with parental responsibilities, gamete donation or sale would not pose any special procreative difficulties.)

d) *Surrogacy:* Surrogacy can involve various kinds of arrangements as to who are the child's biological, gestational, and social parents. For our purposes, we can distinguish between mere gestational surrogacy, where the surrogate gestates another couple's biological child, and surrogacy that involves donor gametes as well as surrogate gestation. Some also distinguish between paid and unpaid surrogacy arrangements.

Pure gestational surrogacy is simply the use of another's uterus for the gestation of a baby. So long as that sort of agreement is free of exploitation, it does not present any distinct procreative moral difficulty. (It can be tricky to navigate the fine line between exploiting surrogates by underpaying them and exploiting them by paying them so much that they agree to be surrogates out of desperation for the money, but that is a general labor issue, and not a problem unique to surrogacy.)

Surrogacy that includes both the use of another's uterus and the use of donor/seller gametes is problematic for the same reasons that it is problematic to donate/sell gametes. Surrogacy arrangements that include donor/seller gametes are also subject to problems regarding responsibility for the resulting pregnancy and child. When the surrogate turns out to be carrying a child with a serious disease or disability, or multiple fetuses when only one was desired, the claim that the commissioning couple are the legal and social parents can become more controversial. Sometimes, an abortion is desired by one party to the arrangement but not another, and agreement cannot be reached.[47] In other surrogacy cases, sometimes when a baby is born disabled, multiple babies are born, or the commissioning couple splits during the pregnancy, one or all parties distance themselves from prior claims of parenthood.[48] These cases point to some of the problems encountered when procreativity is commodified and parental responsibility is assigned vaguely, inconsistently, too diffusely, or not at all. When we add these problems to the problems of widespread exploitation encountered in overseas surrogacy, we note that even those not persuaded by the arguments in Chapter 2 regarding how and when parental responsibility is incurred have many serious problems to overcome before surrogacy can be deemed morally unproblematic.

IV   CONCLUSION

We have seen how our principles might apply to procreative cases. Areas for further research include considering how third-party interests might be incorporated into a broader theory of procreative ethics and population policy.

---

47. See Elizabeth Cohen, "Surrogate Offered $10,000 to Abort Baby," CNN, March 6, 2013, http://www.cnn.com/2013/03/04/health/surrogacy-kelley-legal-battle/.

48. See "Surrogate Mother Left to Care for Biological Parents' Twins," *HuffPost Live*, March 19, 2003; John M. Glionna, "Twins Rejected, Birth Mother Sues," *Los Angeles Times*, August 11, 2001; and Tamar Lewin, "Surrogate Mother Able to Sue for Negligence," *New York Times*, September 20, 1992.

Conclusion

The ideas in this book are intended to help people think through individual procreative choices. I did not discuss implications for law or public policy because law and public policy have to take into account many important factors beyond considering what is a defensible moral choice for an individual. For example, although I argue that adolescent procreation is, barring extraordinary circumstances, morally impermissible, it would not be a good idea to legislate against it. Problems with attempts to legislate who can and cannot procreate include difficulties regarding the legitimacy and potential abuses of power, enforcement, and sanction.

The policy implications of this book are a subject for further study and thought. A few preliminary policies do seem to follow, though, particularly in areas of procreative ethics that are already part of our public legal and medical system. In these areas, public policy already exists, and a more reasoned policy would be an improvement. For example, since I consider gamete donation or sale to be cases of irresponsible procreation, it seems to me that this practice should be abandoned. (At the very least, children of gamete donors should be allowed to know their biological origins, just as adoptees have argued for their right to know theirs.) PGD and similar reproductive technologies should generally be restricted to select for nondiseased embryos. And, finally, the ethics of using experimental reproductive technology should be reviewed and assessed by neutral informed parties, not by those who are deeply enmeshed in a conflict of interests, such as prospective parents and the doctors, hospitals, clinics, and laboratories that stand to profit from the experimental technologies.

I note that having children is one of life's uniquely fulfilling experiences, and it is unfortunate that many people do not have the resources needed to properly raise and nurture a child. The appropriate response to this sad situation, however, is not empty slogans about procreative liberty or any so-called right to have a child. The appropriate response is far more difficult: it is to help people be in a position in which they do have the resources needed to properly raise and nurture a child, and to make the world an easier place for children, and the adults into which they grow, to live in. Instead of treating children as a private luxury, like a yacht you have to pay for all on your own, children ought to be recognized as far more important in and of themselves, and also to adults and to society. If you want more people to be able to permissibly procreate, slogans and easy, lazy, and ultimately pernicious permissions are not going to cut it. You have to change the world.

WORKS CITED

Alloy, L. B. and Abramson, L. Y., "Judgment of Contingency in Depressed and Nondepressed Students: Sadder but Wiser?" *Journal of Experimental Psychology* 1979 108: 441–485.

Alzheimer's Association, "Down Syndrome and Alzheimer's Disease," Alz.org.

Anderson, Elizabeth, "Is Women's Labor a Commodity?" *Philosophy and Public Affairs* 1990 19: 71–92.

Anderson, Elizabeth, *Value in Ethics and Economics*, Harvard University Press, 1993.

Associated Press, "Kansas Man Who Donated Sperm to Lesbian Couple Being Sued by State for Child Support," January 13, 2013.

Barber, J. S., Axinn, W. G., and Thornton, A., "Unwanted Childbearing, Health, and Mother Child Relationships," *Journal of Health and Social Behavior* 1999 40: 231–257.

Baron-Cohen, Simon, *The Science of Evil: On Empathy and the Origins of Cruelty*, Basic Books, 2011.

Bayne, Tim, "Gamete Donation and Parental Responsibility," *Journal of Applied Philosophy* 2003 20: 77–87.

Bayne, Tim, and Kolers, Avery, "Toward a Pluralistic Account of Parenthood," *Bioethics* 2003 17: 221–242.

Belkin, Lisa, "The Made-to-Order Savior," *New York Times*, July 1, 2001.

Belsky, J., "Parental and Nonparental Child Care and Children's Socioeconomic Development: A Decade in Review," *Journal of Marriage and the Family* 1990 52: 885–903.

Benatar, David, *Better Never to Have Been: The Harm of Coming into Existence*, Oxford University Press, 2006.

Benatar, David, "The Unbearable Lightness of Bringing into Being," *Journal of Applied Philosophy* 1999 16: 173–180.

Benatar, David, "Why It Is Better Never to Come into Existence," *American Philosophical Quarterly* 1997 34: 345–355.

Benhabib, Seyla, "Cultural Complexity, Moral Interdependence, and the Global Dialogical Community," Glover, Jonathan, and Nussbaum, Martha, Eds., *Women, Culture, and Development*, Oxford University Press, 1995.

Bloom, Paul, "I'm O.K., You're a Psychopath," *New York Times*, June 17, 2011.

Blum, H. M., Boyle, M. H., and Offord, D. R., "Single Parent Families: Child Psychiatric Disorder and School Performance," *Journal of the American Academy of Child and Adolescent Psychiatry* 1998 27: 214–219.

Blustein, Jeffrey, "Procreation and Parental Responsibility," *Journal of Social Philosophy* 1997 28: 80–82.

Boonin, David, *The Non-identity Problem and the Ethics of Future People*, Oxford University Press, 2014.

Born in Slavery: Slave Narratives from the Federal Writer's Project, 1936–1938, Library of Congress, http://memory.loc.gov/ammem/snhtml/snhome.html.

Brighouse, Harry and Swift, Adam, "Parents' Rights and the Value of the Family," *Ethics* 2006 117: 80–108.

Brodzinsky, David, *The Psychology of Adoption*, Oxford University Press, 1990.

Brownee, Kimberley and Cureton, Adam, Eds., *Disability and Disadvantage*, Oxford University Press, 2009.

Campbell, Angus, Converse, Philip E., and Rogers, Willard L., *The Quality of American Life*, Russell Sage Foundation, 1976.

Camus, Albert, *The Myth of Sisyphus*, Vintage International, 1991.

Carnevale, Anthony P., Rose, Stephen J., and Cheah, Ban, " The College Payoff: Education, Occupations, Lifetime Earnings," *Georgetown University Center on Education and the Workforce*, 2011.

Cohen, Elizabeth, "Surrogate Offered $10,000 to Abort Baby," *CNN*, March 6, 2013.

Collins, Francis, "The Language of Life: DNA and the Revolution" in *Personalised Medicine*, Harper, 2010.

Coogle, Adam, "Saudi Arabia to Women: 'Don't Speak Up, We Know What's Best for You,'" *Daily Beast*.

Craddock, N., and Jones, I., "Genetics of Bipolar Disorder," *Journal of Medical Genetics* 1999 36: 585–594.

Darwall, Stephen, *The Second-Person Standpoint: Morality, Respect, and Accountability*, Harvard University Press, 2009.

Davidowitz, Lucy, *The War against the Jews: 1933–1945*, Bantam, 1975.

Dayal, Molina B., Lucidi, Richard Scott, et al., "Preimplantation Genetic Diagnosis," *Medscape Reference*, August 29, 2013, http://emedicine.medscape.com/article/273415- overview#aw2aab6b4.

DeGrazia, David, *Creation Ethics: Reproduction, Genetics, and Quality of Life*, Oxford University Press, 2012.

DeParle, Jason, "Two Classes, Divided by 'I Do,'" *New York Times*, July 14, 2012.

Diener, Ed, and Diener, Carol, "Most People Are Happy," *Psychological Science* 1996 7: 181–185.

Diener, Ed, et al., "Subjective Well-Being: Three Decades of Progress," *Psychological Bulletin* 1999 125: 276–302.

Diener, Marissa, and McGavran, Mary Beth Diener, "What Makes People Happy? A Developmental Approach to the Literature on Family Relationships and Well-Being," *The Science of Subjective Well-Being*, Eid, Michael, and Larson, Randy J, Eds., Guilford Press, 2008.

Dobson, K., and Franche, R. L., "A Conceptual and Empirical Review of the Depressive Realism Hypothesis," *Canadian Journal of Behavioural Science* 1989 21: 419–433.

D'Onofrio, Brian M., Rickert, Martin E., et al., "Paternal Age at Childbearing and Offspring Psychiatric and Academic Morbidity," *JAMA Psychiatry*, online first, February 26, 2014.

Douglass, Frederick, *Narrative of the Life of Frederick Douglass*, Bedford / St. Martin's, 2002.

Dworkin, Ronald, "Paternalism," *Monist* 1972 56: 64–84.

Dworkin, Ronald, "The Original Position," *University of Chicago Law Review* 1973 40: 500–533.

Feinberg, Joel, "The Child's Right to an Open Future," *Whose Child? Children's Rights, Parental Authority, and State Power*, Aiken, William, and LaFollette, Hugh, Eds., Littlefield, Adams, 1980.

Feinberg, Joel, "Wrongful Life and the Counterfactual Element in Harming," *Social Philosophy and Policy* 1986 4: 145–179.

Feldman, Fred, *Confrontations with the Reaper*, Oxford University Press, 1992.

Feldman, Susan, "Multiple Biological Mothers: The Case for Gestation," *Journal of Social Philosophy* 1992 23: 98–104.

Finkel, Eli J., and Fitzsimons, Grainne M., "When Helping Hurts," *New York Times*, May 10, 2013.

Fisch, H., Hyun, G., et al., "The Influence of Paternal Age on Down syndrome," *Journal of Urology* 2003 169: 2275–2278.

Fox-Genovese, Elizabeth, *Within the Plantation Household: Black and White Women in the Old South*, University of North Carolina Press, 1988.

Frankl, Victor, *Man's Search for Meaning*, Hogger and Stoughton, 1971.

Frey, Rebecca, "Genetic Factors and Mental Disorders," *Encyclopedia of Mental Disorders*, web: http://www.minddisorders.com/Flu-Inv/Genetic-factors-and-mentaldisorders.html.

Friedrich, Daniel, "A Duty to Adopt?" *Journal of Applied Philosophy* 2013 30: 25–39.

Giuliana Fuscaldo, "Genetic Ties: Are They Morally Binding?" *Bioethics* 2006 20: 64–76.

Gallagher, Maggie, "What Is Marriage For? The Public Purposes of Marriage Law," *Louisiana Law Review* 2001–2002 62: 773– 791.

Gelles, Richard, "Child Abuse and Violence in Single-Parent Families: Parent Absence and Economic Deprivation," *American Journal of Orthopsychiatry* 1989 59: 492–501.

Glionna, John M., "Twins Rejected, Birth Mother Sues," *Los Angeles Times*, August 11, 2001.

Glover, Jonathan, *Choosing Children: Genes, Disability, and Design*, Oxford University Press, 2006.

Golomb, Elan, *Trapped in the Mirror: Adult Children of Narcissists in Their Struggle for Self*, William Morrow, 1992.

Hanser, Matthew, "Harming Future People," *Philosophy and Public Affairs* 1990 19: 47–70.

Hare, Caspar, "Voices from Another World: Must We Respect the Interests of People Who Do Not, and Will Never, Exist?" *Ethics* 2007 117: 498–523.

Hare, R. M., "Rawls' Theory of Justice," *Reading Rawls*, Daniels, Norman, Ed., Stanford University Press, 1989.

Harman, Elizabeth, "Can We Harm and Benefit in Creating?" *Philosophical Perspectives* 2004 18: 89–109.

Haugaard, J. J., Schustack, A., et al., "Birth Mothers Who Voluntarily Relinquish Infants for Adoption," *Adoption Quarterly* 1998 2: 89–97.

Herzog, Don, *Happy Slaves*, University of Chicago Press, 1989.

Hill, J. L., "'What Does It Mean to Be a Parent?': The Claims of Biology as the Basis for Parental Rights," *New York University Law Review* 1991 66: 353–420.

Hirvelä, Shari, and Helkama, Klaus, "Empathy, Values, Morality, and Asperger's Syndrome," *Scandinavian Journal of Psychology* 2011 52: 560–572.

Hook, Ernest B., Cross, Phillip K., and Schreinemachers, Dina M., "Chromosomal Abnormality Rates at Amniocentesis and in Live-Born Infants," *Journal of the American Medical Association* 1983 249: 2034–2038.

Howe, David, "Attachment: Assessing Children's Needs and Parenting Capacity," *The Child's World: The Comprehensive Guide to Assessing Children in Need*, 2nd edition, Jessica Kingsley Publishers, 2010.

Human Rights Watch, June 26, 2013, http://www.hrw.org/news/2013/06/26/ saudi-arabia-women-dont-speak-we-know-whats-best-you.

HuffPost Live, "Surrogate Mother Left to Care for Biological Parents' Twins," March 19, 2003.

Hurley, Paul, and Weinberg, Rivka, "Whose Problem Is Non-identity?" *Journal of Moral Philosophy*, forthcoming.

In the Matter of Baby M 109 N.J. 396, 537 A. 2nd (N.J. 1988).

Iacopino, Vincent, "The Taliban's War on Women," report for *Physicians for Human Rights*, http://physiciansforhumanrights.org/library/reports/talibans-war-on-women-1998.html.

Jones, Adele, "Issues Relevant to Therapy with Adoptees," *Psychotherapy: Theory, Research, Practice, Training* 1997 34: 64–68.

Johns Hopkins Health Library entry on schizophrenia: www. hopkinsmedicine. org/healthlibrary/conditions/mental_health_disorders/schizophrenia_85,P00762/

Kant, Immanuel, *Groundwork of the Metaphysics of Morals.*

Kavka, Gregory, "The Paradox of Future Individuals," *Philosophy and Public Affairs* 1981 11: 93–112.

Karnein, Anja J., *A Theory of Unborn Life: From Abortion to Genetic Manipulation*, Oxford University Press, 2012.

Kelland, Kate, "Some Forms of IVF Linked to Rise of Autism, Mental Disability," *Reuters International*, July 2, 2013.

Keller, Matthew, and Nesse, Randolph, "Is Low Mood an Adaptation? Evidence for Subtypes with Symptoms That Match Precipitants," *Journal of Affective Disorders* 2005 86: 27–35.

Kristiansen, Kristjana and Shakespeare, Tom, Eds., *Arguing about Disability: Philosophical Perspectives*, Routledge, 2010.

Lahr, John, "The Disappearing Act," *The New Yorker*, February 2, 2007.

Lanzmann, Claude, director, *Shoah*, 1985.

Leahy, Robert, "Pessimism and the Evolution of Negativity," *Journal of Cognitive Psychotherapy* 2002 16: 295–316.

Lehrer, John, "Depression's Upside," *New York Times*, February 28, 2010.

LeMoyne, Terri, and Buchanan, Tom, "Does Hovering Matter? Helicopter Parenting and Its Effect on Well-Being," *Sociological Spectrum* 2011 31: 399–418.

Lewin, Tamar, "Surrogate Mother Able to Sue for Negligence," *New York Times*, September 20, 1992.

Lowenstein, Sophie, "An Overview of the Concept of Narcissism," *Social Casework* 1997 58: 136– 142.

McCeer, Victoria, "Varieties of Moral Agency: Lessons from Autism (and Psychopathy)," *Moral Psychology*, vol. 3: The Neuroscience of Morality: Emotion, Brain Disorders, and Development, Sinnott-Armstrong, Walter, Ed., MIT Press, 2008.

McLaughlin, Zeanah, et al., "Attachment as a Mechanism Linking Foster Care Placement to Improved Mental Health Outcomes in Previously Institutionalized Children," *Journal of Child Psychology and Psychiatry* 2012 53: 46–55.

McMahan, Jeff, "Problems of Population Theory," *Ethics* 1981 92: 104–107.

McMahan, Jeff, *The Ethics of Killing: Problems at the Margins of Life*, Oxford University Press, 2002.

McMahan, Jeff, "Wrongful Life: Paradoxes in the Morality of Causing People to Exist," *Rational Commitment and Social Justice*, Jules L. Coleman and Christopher W. Morris, Eds., Cambridge University Press, 1998.

Mayohealth.com

Medline Plus, "Huntington's Disease," web.

Mariano, Timothy Y., Chan, Heng Choon (Oliver), and Myers, Wade C., "Toward a More Holistic Understanding of Filicide: A Multidisciplinary Analysis of 32 Years of U.S. Arrest Data," *Forensic Science International* 2014 236: 46–53.

Matlin, Margaret W., and Stang, David J., *The Pollyanna Principle: Selectivity in Language, Memory and Thought*, Schenkman, 1978.

Meyers, David G., and Diener, Ed, "The Pursuit of Happiness," *Scientific American* 1996 274: 70–72.

Mowry, Briana, "Is Being Childfree by Choice Selfish?" *Redbook Magazine*, redbookmag.com/love-sex/advice/childfree-by-choice.

Munson, Ronald, "Artificial Insemination and Donor Responsibility," *Intention and Reflection: Basic Issues in Bioethics*, Wadsworth, 1988.

Nagel, Thomas, "Rawls on Justice," *Philosophical Review* 1973 82: 220–234.

Narayan, Uma, "Family Ties: Rethinking Parental Claims in the Light of Surrogacy and Custody," *Having and Raising Children: Unconventional Families, Hard Choices, and the Social Good*, Narayan, Uma and Bartkowiak, Julia J., Eds., Pennsylvania State University Press, 1999.

Narveson, Jan, "Utilitarianism and New Generations," *Mind* 1967 76: 62–72.

Narverson, Jan, "Moral Problems of Population," *Monist* 1973 57: 62–86.

Lindemann-Nelson, James, "Parental Obligations and the Ethics of Surrogacy: A Causal Perspective," *Public Affairs Quarterly* 1991 5: 49–61.

New York Times, December 2, 1986, "Major Personality Study Finds That Traits Are Mostly Inherited."

New York Times In-Depth report on schizophrenia, web.

Nickman, S. L., and Rosenfeld, A., "Children in Adoptive Families: Overview and Update," *Journal of the Academy of Child and Adolescent Psychiatry* 2005 44: 987–995.

Nozick, Robert, *Anarchy, State, and Utopia*, Basic Books, 1974.

Nussbaum, Martha, "Human Capabilities, Female Human Beings," *Women, Culture, and Development*, Glover, Jonathan, and Nussbaum, Martha, Eds., Oxford University Press, 1995.

O'Connor, Joe, "Trend of Couples Not Having Children Is Just Plain Selfish," *National Post*, September 19, 2012.

O'Neal, Onora, "Between Consenting Adults," *Philosophy and Public Affairs* 1985 14: 252–277.

Olausson, P. O., Cnattingius, S., et al., "Teenage Pregnancies and the Risk of Late Fetal Death and Infant Mortality," *British Journal of Obstetrics and Gynecology* 1999 106: 116–121.

Oremus, Will, "Did Early Christians Practice Birth Control?" *Slate*, February 10, 2012, slate.com/articles/news_and_politics/explainer/2012/02/ obama_birth_control_battle_when_did_catholics_ban_contraception_. html?wpisrc = slate_river.

Overall, Christine, *Why Have Children?* MIT Press, 2012.

Page, Edgar, "Donation, Surrogacy, and Adoption," *Journal of Applied Philosophy* 1985 2: 161–172.

Parfit, Derek, "Comments on the Non-Identity Problem," *Ethics* 1986 96: 832–863.

Parfit, Derek, "Future Generations, Further Problems," *Philosophy and Public Affairs* 1982 11: 113–172.

Parfit, Derek, *On What Matters*, Oxford University Press, 2011.

Parfit, Derek, *Reasons and Persons*, Oxford University Press, 1984.

Phipps, Maureen G., Sowers, Maryfran, et al., "The Risk for Infant Mortality among Adolescent Chilbearing Groups," *Journal of Women's Health* 2002 11: 889–897.

Rawls, John, *A Theory of Justice*, Harvard University Press, 1971.

Reich, Annie, "Pathological Forms of Self-Esteem Regulation," *Psychoanalytic Study of the Child* 1960 15: 215–232.

Ripstein, Arthur, *Equality, Responsibility, and the Law*, Cambridge University Press, 1996.

Ripstein, Arthur, *Force and Freedom*, Harvard University Press, 2009.

Roberts, Melinda, *Child versus Childmaker*, Rowman & Littlefield, 1998.

Roberts, Melinda, "Good Intentions and a Great Divide: Having Babies by Intending Them," *Law and Philosophy* 1983 12: 287–317.

Robertson, John, *Children of Choice: Freedom and the New Reproductive Technologies*, Princeton University Press, 1994.

Roberstson, John, "Procreative Liberty and Harm to Offspring in Assisted Reproduction," *American Journal of Law and Medicine* 2004 30: 7–40.

Rothman, Barbara, *Recreating Motherhood: Ideology and Technology in a Patriarchal Society*, Norton, 1989.

Sack, W. H., Mason, R., and Higgins, J. E., "The Single-Parent Family and Abusive Child Punishment," *American Journal of Orthopsychiatry* 1985 55: 252–259.

Sandel, Michael, *The Case against Perfection*, Harvard University Press, 2007.

Savulescu, Julian, and Kahane, Guy, "The Moral Obligation to Create Children with the Best Chance of the Best Life," *Bioethics* 2009 23: 274–290.

Scanlon, T. M., *What We Owe To Each Other*, Harvard University Press, 1998.

Sen, Amartya, *Commodities and Capabilities*, Oxford University Press, 1985.

Schiffrin, Holly H., Liss, Miriam, et al., "Helping or Hovering? The Effects of Helicopter Parenting on College Students' Well-Being," *Journal of Child and Family Studies*, February 9, 2013.

Shiffrin, Seana, "Wrongful Life, Procreative Responsibility, and the Significance of Harm," *Legal Theory* 1999 5: 117–148.

Skaine, Rosemarie, *The Women of Afghanistan under the Taliban*, McFarland, 2002.

Solomon, Andrew, *Far from the Tree*, Scribner / Simon & Schuster, 2012.

Smilansky, Saul, "Is There a Moral Obligation to Have Children?" *Journal of Applied Philosophy* 1995 12: 41–53.

Smilansky, Saul, "Life Is Good," *South African Journal of Philosophy* 2012 31: 69–78.

Smilansky, Saul, "Preferring Not to Have Been Born," *10 Moral Paradoxes*, WileyBlackwell, 2007.

Solomon, Judith, and George, Carol, "The Disorganized Attachment Caregiving System: Disregulation of Adaptive Processes at Multiple Levels," *Disorganized Attachment and Caregiving*, Solomon, Judith, and George, Carol, Eds., Guilford Press, 2011.

Sperling, Daniel, *Posthumous Interests*, Cambridge University Press, 2008.

Steinbock, Bonnie, "The Logical Case for Wrongful Life," *Hastings Center Report* 1986 16: 15–20.

Stewart, Janet, "Down Syndrome/Trisomy 21," *Genetic Drift: Management of Common Genetic Disorders*, 1998 16.

Sunstein, Cass, "Preferences and Politics," *Philosophy and Public Affairs* 1991 20: 3–34.

Sunstein, Cass R., and Thaler, Richard H. "Libertarian Paternalism Is Not an Oxymoron," *University of Chicago Law Review* 2003 70: 1159–1206.

Tellegen, Auke, Lykken, David, et al., "Personality Similarity in Twins Reared Apart and Together," *Journal of Personality and Social Psychology* 1988 54: 1031–1039.

Tuomela, Raimo and Miller, Kaarlo, "We-Intentions," *Philosophical Studies* 1988 53: 367–389.

Uher, R., "The Role of Genetic Variation in the Causation of Mental Illness: An Evolution-Informed Framework," *Mollecular Psychiatry* 2009 14: 1072–1082.

The University of Southern California Shoah Foundation archives, http://sfi.usc.edu/.

Velleman, David, "Love and Nonexistence," *Philosophy and Public Affairs* 2008 36: 266–288

Velleman, David, "The Gift of Life," *Philosophy and Public Affairs* 2008 36: 245–266.

Velleman, David, "Well Being and Time," *Pacific Philosophical Quarterly* 1991 72: 48–71.

Wasserman, David, "The Non-identity Problem, Disability, and the Role Morality of Prospective Parents," *Ethics* 2005 116: 132–152.

Weinberg, Rivka, "Existence: Who Needs It? The Non-identity Problem and Merely Possible People," *Bioethics* 2013 27: 471–484.

Weinberg, Rivka, "Identifying and Dissolving the Non-identity Problem," *Philosophical Studies* 2008 137: 3–18.

Weinberg, Rivka "Is Having Children Always Wrong?" *South African Journal of Philosophy* 2012 31: 26–37.

Weinberg, Rivka, "Procreative Justice: A Contractualist Account," *Public Affairs Quarterly* 2002 16: 405–425.

Weinberg, Rivka, "The Moral Complexity of Sperm Donation," *Bioethics* 2008 22: 166–178.

Weinreb, Maxine, and Murphy, Bianca, "The Birth Mother," *Women and Therapy* 1988 7: 23–36.

Wieseltier, Leon, *Kaddish*, Vintage Books / Random House, 1998.

Williams, Bernard, "A Critique of Utilitarianism," *Utilitarianism For and Against*, Smart, J. J. C., and Williams, Bernard, Cambridge University Press, 1973.

Wolf, Susan, *Meaning in Life and Why It Matters*, Princeton University Press, 2010.

Woodward, James, "The Non-identity Problem," *Ethics* 1986 96: 805–831.

Woodward, James, "Reply to Parfit's 'Comments on the Non-Identity Problem,'" *Ethics* 1987 97: 800–816.

Wilson, Robin Fretwell, "Evaluating Marriage: Does Marriage Matter to the Nurturing of Children?" *San Diego Law Review* 2005 42: 847–881.

INDEX